# Staying Sane™
## When You're
# DIETING

# Staying Sane™

# When You're

# DIETING

*Pamela K. Brodowsky*
*Evelyn M. Fazio*

Da Capo
LIFE
LONG

A Member of the Perseus Books Group

Set in 12-point New Baskerville by the Perseus Books Group

Library of Congress Cataloging-in-Publication Data
Brodowsky, Pamela K.
    Staying sane when you're dieting / Pamela K. Brodowsky, Evelyn M. Fazio.—
1st Da Capo Press ed.
      p.   cm. — (Staying sane series)
    ISBN-13: 978-0-7382-1035-3 (isbn-13; pbk. : alk. paper)
    ISBN-10: 0-7382-1035-8 (isbn-10; pbk. : alk. paper)
    1. Weight loss—Psychological aspects—Popular works.   I. Fazio, Evelyn M.
II. Title.   III. Series.
    RM222.2.B7814   2005
    613.2'5'019—dc22

2005020418

First Da Capo Press edition 2005

Published by Da Capo Press
A Member of the Perseus Books Group
www.dacapopress.com

Da Capo Press books are available at special discounts for bulk purchases in the U.S. by corporations, institutions, and other organizations. For more information, please contact the Special Markets Department at the Perseus Books Group, 11 Cambridge Center, Cambridge, MA 02142, or call (800) 255-1514 or (617) 252-5298, or e-mail special.markets@perseusbooks.com.

1 2 3 4 5 6 7 8 9—08 07 06 05

To our partner in crime, Marnie Cochran,
executive editor at Da Capo Press,
for her encouragement, help, and enthusiasm
for the Staying Sane™ series.

# Contents

## 1 When You Have Diet Temptations, Downfalls, and Disasters

## 2 When You're on a Brand-Name Diet

# 3  When You Cheat on Your Diet    47

# 4  When You Design Your Own Diet    63

## 8　When Your Diet Drives Everyone Else Crazy　167

## 9　When You Have Dieting Helpers　183

## 10　When Your Diet Is Frustrating You　193

# About the Staying Sane Series

The Staying Sane series is a collection of funny, irreverent, light-hearted, yet sassy, advice-laden books that are dedicated to finding the silver lining in the annoying, frustrating, or trying situations we all encounter every day.

The Staying Sane series shows you how to look for—and find—the humor and enlightenment in nearly every situation—you need only to be open to seeing it. Let's face it: We all experience difficult times in our lives, and that's precisely why we've developed the Staying Sane series.

We want you to know that we've been through all kinds of demented things ourselves (oh, have we ever!), and we and our contributors plan to focus each volume on a specific topic to help you cope with some of the most typical—and most common—situations we all face at one point or another as we try to get through life.

The Staying Sane series' intention is to shed light on difficult situations, to bring laughter to people who are caught in a web of frustration and petty annoyances, and to provide help, advice and answers in every situation;—at the same time, we want to let readers know that they are not the only ones who've suffered through these trying, irritating episodes or situations. As laughter is truly the best medicine, the Staying Sane series will help you get through whatever comes up with as few dents and bruises as possible, and, we hope, with your family relationships and friendships still intact when all is said (or not) and done (or not!).

Just hearing about other people's problems usually makes our own seem trivial by comparison, making us realize that things aren't really so bad. What's more, by reading about the scores of other people who've had the same or worse experience, we are able to get a more realistic perspective and regain our sense of proportion—all because we've been able to step back and see that things really could be much worse. And besides, misery loves company, doesn't it?

Staying sane it isn't as hard as you think. Keeping it together when all hell breaks loose is just part of life—

something we have to do every day if we're living on planet Earth.

But one thing to keep in mind is that there is always someone else out there who is also on the edge of losing it. Our lives are complicated, but this doesn't mean we can't laugh at our problems—it can really help make them seem smaller and less overwhelming.

So when things are getting out of hand and you just don't think you can take it anymore, pick up a copy of one of the Staying Sane titles. It may be just what you need to keep from going off the deep end. We'll be right there with you, helping you cope!

## Let Us Know

We would be delighted to hear your reactions to the stories in this and all Staying Sane books. Please let us know which stories you liked the most and how they related to your life.

Please send us your stories for upcoming volumes of the Staying Sane series. Our email address is:

submission@staying-sane.com

You can also visit us on the Web at:

www.staying-sane.com

We look forward to hearing from you!

*Pam and Evelyn*

# About *Staying Sane* *When You're Dieting*

Let's face it—dieting isn't fun. It's something that we all hate doing, but we find ourselves needing to diet for a variety of reasons. Whether it's because the doctor insists upon it, your high school reunion is coming up and you want to wear the same size dress as you wore twenty-five years ago, you're going to a family event and want to look your best, or your daughter is getting married and your ex-husband will be there with his trophy wife and you need to look like a goddess so that he eats his heart out for the rest of eternity, it's going to be an annoyance and an inconvenience to have to think about what you eat until you're slinky and slim.

We've all been there and done that. We've all tried to wiggle our fat butts into clothes that are too tight, struggled to get our jeans up over our ever-spreading hips, or dreaded putting on a swimsuit for the first time each summer. Some of us have even had trouble getting our shoes over our fat feet. (Whatever the situation, nobody—and we mean *nobody,* ever wants to give up that second helping of dinner, or that tasty dessert, but that's what's in store for you when you're on a diet.

Rather than try to sugar-coat the experience, we're going to level with you. You have to make up your mind, get a grip, and do what's needed so that you can get where you need to go: down a size or two, or a lot more if it's necessary.

Before we begin, let's find out how badly you need the advice we're about to impart. Take the following quiz and see where you stand:

## SANITY QUIZ

1. Does the mere idea of going on a diet make you break out in hives?
2. Do you find yourself sneaking food in the middle of the night?
3. Do you snack all day long, then try to hide it?

4. Is your partner always on your back about your eating habits?
5. Are you addicted to sweets?
6. Do you crave certain foods while dieting?
7. Are you so embarrassed by your size and shape that you hate looking in the mirror?
8. Do you find yourself gaining when you're supposed to be losing?
9. Do you wish you looked the way you used to look?
10. Do you think dieting is just a waste of time?

If you answered yes to even one of these questions, then *Staying Sane When You're Dieting* is the book for you. Here you'll find useful advice along with hilarious stories right from the trenches, from people just like you, who needed to diet and survived to meet their goals. Whether they dieted with partners or on their own, whether they made up their own brand of diet or followed a well-known plan, these folks know the ropes and will help you get over that big fat hump!

So sit down with your glass of water and your lemon slice, or your cup of green tea with kombucha, or whatever happens to be your dieting beverage du jour, and read on. Find out how our contributors coped with dieting; they'll give you all their best secrets and advice to help you reach your dieting goals as pleasantly and painlessly as possible. You'll get plenty of laughs along the way, and although we won't be there to watch you get on the scale, we'll be cheering you on from the sidelines. We've been there, we've done that, and we know exactly what you're going through!

# 1

# When You Have Diet Temptations, Downfalls, and Disasters

## Fat Tuesday
Edward F. Fitzgerald

## Other People's Dinners
Joyce Romano

## Hershey: Or Dieting Isn't Sane
Ray Zardetto

# Sanity Quiz

You have tried everything to lose weight and nothing seems to work. Your problem stems from your delight in snacking. You are a habitual snack attacker. You can't bring yourself to pass up anything sweet on the road to success. Today is your office holiday party. The tables are full of mouth watering delights. However, just yesterday you overheard your coworkers talking about your ever increasing girth and newfound expansion, especially in the middle and hindquarters.

Do you

A. eat all you want
B. shovel as much in as you can while no one is looking
C. pack as many crab cakes and baby lamb chops as you can into a party napkin and shove them into your pockets so that nobody will know
D. all of the above

If you answered yes to any of these questions, then you need to check out the stories and advice to come. Just wait and see how these folks survived their own dieting disasters and lived to tell the tale.

# Fat Tuesday

*Edward F. Fitzgerald*

THE SCREAM DID IT.

Woke me and the cats.

Four a.m., and I'm bolting out of bed, racing toward the kitchen, skidding over two panicked fur balls at the first turn, tumbling head-first over a third, and sliding across the tiles into the kitchen.

I didn't blame the cats. It's every man and beast for himself.

We knew. My wife, stumbling half-asleep into the bathroom, had stepped onto that damnable scale!

Thus the screech heard round the world.

It was definitely Fat Tuesday.

In seconds I was at the refrigerator shoving a hunk of cheesecake into my mouth and grabbing for caramels as if they were going out of style. Which they were. Before the door slammed shut, catching my PJs in the rubber seal and flattening me along its edge like a spotted-gecko, Pittypat, my very own Significant Wife, had arrived.

"How *can* you eat that vile, disgusting, *fattening* crap?" she hissed.

A karate-chop to my wrist sent caramels a-scatter. A grab at the short hairs at the nape of my neck (which, I suppose, was preferable to another choice that comes to mind), and I was spun into the room, five knowing cats peering down nervously from our pot shelves. Pittypat pulled the kitchen trash bin close, her eyes like radar wands as they scanned the brightly-lit contents of the sacred cold cabinet.

"Enough is enough," she growled, sharpish teeth disfiguring her pretty lips. "Bring another trash bin," she added, "This one won't half do."

*Gone*—the rest of the cheesecake that only yesterday she had lovingly spooned into my bird-like mouth. *Gone*—the caramels, a barely opened gallon of ice cream, the half-and-half, the chocolate turtles (her fingerprint still embedded in one), the English muffins, the white bread, the gourmet cookies. Even the buttered string beans with almonds.

*Gone*—pot roast leftovers, a pound of bacon—disappearing too fast for the eye to follow. And her muttered imprecations, only parts of which I dare repeat. "*Cheesecake?* Are we mad? Have we gone entirely insane? *Caramels?* How *old* are you, anyway, Chub? *Beef!* Beef *sucks!* Name of God, *everyone* knows that! *Butter!* Sure! Let's run over to the cardiac ward and eat it there so you can be ready when the clots hit."

A smart chess player simply tips over his king and resigns when the game is beyond recovery. I played my role without prompting. Bringing more trash bins and watching despondently as the best of Trader Joe's headed for the Mesa landfill. Farewell! I tried to adhere to George M. Cohan's plea, "Always leave them laughing when you say goodbye," but it was more than I could manage.

And what, indeed, was the triggering event for this Rape of the Pralines?

Well, we know that Pittypat stepped onto the scale, of course, but to what effect? Had a mysterious forty pounds suddenly materialized? Had she fallen and found herself unable to rise, the helpless captive of an unexpectedly expanded middle?

Let's put this in perspective.

Pittypat stands five feet two inches and weighs 110 pounds!

That's *before* she's dried off after showering. She's a mere slip!

Bent over grasping her ankles, you could mail her anywhere, FedEx® priority pack. Forget your house-key? She'll slide in under the door. Are you getting the picture? Did I say 110 pounds give or take? We have to allow a *little* play in the fateful numbers, surely.

Occasionally, when she's been very active, Pittypat will actually drop a pound or three, which, I hasten to add, she can ill afford to do. (In truth, that has on occasion saved us X-ray money—when the doctor, by chance, has positioned her against a strong light.) On the fateful morning of which I am now reporting, however, the needle swayed in the other direction. Oh, woe! Aye, woe, I say, to all within reach, my friends, when the arrow moves up.

"*Look* at this," she'll wail, pinching a quarter-centimeter of wayward flesh between two fingers. "This is disgusting! Why didn't you tell me I was getting fat? Didn't you *notice?*"

*Uh-oh! Hit the lifeboats, men! Abandon ship. Now hear this! Do not answer! Do not answer! Launch flares and row for shore!*

"Honey, I don't care what that scale says. You are not fat. I'm looking at you right now and you look beautiful."

*All obesity-attack survivors fall out on the quarterdeck for the awarding of medals! You, the guy who said, "You look beautiful," come up here in front.*

Of course, when these fat-attacks do hit, they are kamikaze specials heading for the smokestacks of the battleship life. Sweets and goodies, cream and butter, even red meat—gone! White meat—well, maybe— *once in a great while.*

It's Brussels sprouts time, folks—those dwarfish cabbages that cause rats to leave shore and return to the sinking ship. Spinach salads. Broccoli in yellow barf-sauce. Low-fat yogurt and veggie delights. Shredded hemp lying atop God knows what. Carrot sticks until your skin turns mango-orange and jaundiced alcoholics look upon you in envy. And white glop thrown from a trowel onto your plate.

It's hard to explain, really, the unreasoning panic that overtakes us when we are confronted by the ogre of weight gain. It doesn't matter a whit that she is a female who rarely strays above 110 pounds. If the "number" passes 110—that's it, Baby! The yawning pit of obesity beckons.

Believe me, that miserable deus ex machina in the bathroom doesn't help. And my description is apt because that vile scale is indeed a contrived solution for what we all believe to be an insoluble difficulty (keeping our weight at the "right" number).

*You ran the decathlon last week? You came in third in the "tough man" race?*

Pish tosh! Let's have the number, Chub? What does the sainted box say today?

Okay, as a nation, we are obese. True. Our grade school kids now look like Rose Bowl floats marching into class. But must we adults become slaves to the prattling of talk-show gurus and exercise freaks? Hostage to calorie charts originally designed by Sacher Masoch? (Incidentally, that original masochist got his green card and now works for the Arizona Department of Health as a taco-taster, so he gets all the pain he can handle.)

Take me, for example. Should I worry if my weight creeps up a pound or two? At 212 pounds, I am an acceptable weight for a male who stands six feet one inch, don't you agree? Well, alright, I'm only five feet seven, which in fact might suggest a teeny problem, but, let's keep our heads.

First, liposuction is a sucky solution (literally and figuratively), and a tube-fed diet of oatmeal and prune juice is unnecessarily extreme. Instead, I propose the following eminently reasonable weight-loss plan, and I ask only that readers of *Staying Sane* vote to approve it. Send your letters and emails immediately. If approved, I propose to do the following:

*Study the Problem Thoroughly.* I will read the 114 books on dieting that we have purchased, and also the seventy-three books and pamphlets from Pittypat's mother (excluding *Witchcraft Will Make You Thin,* her autobiography). I will make copious notes as well as a chart in six colors to cover our living room wall—a terrific conversation piece when Pittypat has her celery-sniffing friends over for a low-cal snack.

*Eat Smaller Portions.* A typical lunch would be a lean hamburger patty, a thin slice of cheese, three little pickles, a tiny pat of butter on my little bitty roll, a tablespoon of mayo, a tiny wallop of Russian dressing, a junior mocha milkshake, and a miniscule piece of apple strudel with just enough ice cream to make it slide down easily. What could be more reasonable than that—and still keep our struggling economy flourishing, eh? (If a man is not a patriot, what good is he?)

*Exercise Vigorously.* I will hang up my old punching bag in the garage and strike it weekly (on trash day as I put out our barrels). I will place my large barbell and weights in the middle of the living room floor where I can study them. I will pull the taped leaf-bags off the treadmill. I will sort through the rest of the $16,575 worth of exercise equipment that I have purchased over the last three years and pick at least one item that would look nice sitting beside the treadmill.

*Walk, Walk, Walk!*   I will walk everywhere! From our bed to the toilet, from the bedroom to the kitchen, from the kitchen to the living room and back to the kitchen, *and out to the car*—everywhere! And last, a critical part of my plan, I will *take a sledge and smash that back-stabbing landmine in the bathroom into a million pieces!*

Well, don't just sit there, dammit! Vote!

Edward F. Fitzgerald is the author of *Bank's Bandits: The Untold Story of The Original Green Berets,* and a law textbook published by Westlaw.

# Other People's Dinners

*Joyce Romano*

WE DECIDED TO RISK IT ALL . . . because we were poor, we were hungry, we were college students.

On our way home from one of our crazy road trips, my guy friends wanted to stop for a bite to eat. There weren't a lot of dining choices on that country road. We finally fell upon a nice restaurant that looked good, although a little pricey for starving students. I didn't want to go, I really didn't. I was on a diet after all, and this restaurant probably had really good food. How could I possibly resist all the mouth-watering temptations? Well, easy enough. I had only enough money for a side salad—maybe.

I should have known this night would turn out to be an adventure; after all, every night out with Henry, Artie, and John was entertaining. These wild and crazy guys were fun; they were big healthy athletic guys who lived life to the fullest. And they ate like sumo wrestlers at fast-food joints. But they, too, were poor college students and at this restaurant they would have to fill up on French fries and gravy, vanilla cokes, and Saltine crackers.

We gave our simple orders to the waiter. While waiting for our food, we couldn't help but overhear the argument going on between an older couple in the booth across from ours. They were bickering so much that they didn't even pay attention when the waiter brought their platters filled with lobster, crab legs, and crusty garlic bread. They just got louder and angrier with one another.

I noticed that while their argument escalated they didn't touch their food. My hungry friends and I were forced to eat the cheapest things on the menu only to endure the delicious scents of seafood and drawn butter wafting at us from the other table. But I consoled myself by knowing that I was sticking to my diet.

Moments later, our meager meals came. As we started eating, I glanced over as the woman at the next table got up. She slapped her partner's face and ran out of the restaurant. Of course, everyone in the restaurant was looking now. The poor guy just sat there with his head down and licked his wounds.

Embarrassed for him, we looked away and went back to our conversation and our "snack." A few minutes later, the guy got up and ran out of the restaurant. Henry said, "Wow, their dinner is getting cold." That's Henry for you, more concerned about the food than the rocky romance.

Minutes passed . . . five minutes . . . ten minutes. The lobster and crab legs just sat there untouched.

The same realization hit all of us at the same moment: These people weren't coming back!

Finally, Artie said, "It's a sin to waste that lobster. Henry, go grab it before the busboy comes and takes it away."

Henry looked horrified and said, "Why me? You go get it, Artie, what do I look like?"

"You look hungry, just like the rest of us and that lobster is calling our name and you *are* on the aisle," Artie said.

After another minute, Henry glanced around the restaurant to make sure the coast was clear, got up, and grabbed the platters and brought them to our table of hungry jackals. The guys dug in. The food smelled great. It looked great. My salad hadn't even put a dent in my appetite. But I couldn't blow the diet.

"Have some," said Artie.

"But I'm on a diet," said I.

"Oh, go on and eat," said John.

"I need to stay on my diet," said I.

"It's sooooo good!" said Artie.

"But, but . . . my diet," said I.

"Screw the diet," said Henry.

"Easy for you guys. You aren't chubby," said I.

"Be quiet and eat," all three said.

After another minute of listening to the lusty sounds of my friends' delirious enjoyment of the free food, I finally gave in. I threw caution and the diet to the wind. Just as I was about to break open my first crab leg and dip it deep into the thick sensual butter sauce, John let out a desperate whisper, "Oh, dear God, no!"

"Oh dear God, no, what?" I asked.

John just stared bug-eyed down the aisle. We all turned and looked. The couple were on their way back to the table. Oh dear God, no! They were gone fifteen minutes; we thought they were gone for good. Or maybe in our hunger and our desire to eat free lobster, it seemed like fifteen minutes, but there was no doubt now . . . they were coming back to their table. We looked at each in horror. Now what should we do?

"Quick, start stuffing the lobster and crab legs down your shirt," yelled John. We stared at him as he stuffed crab legs in his shirt. We looked at each other, and after two heartbeats we started frantically grabbing and shoving legs into our clothing, which, believe me, is not easy to do when you are in a rush.

We were a frenzy of motion and words. "Hurry, sit on the plates!" "Grab the garlic bread and eat it!" "Put those plates on the floor!" "Hurry, hurry, hurry!"

Seconds later, as we sat there with spiny sea legs pinching our skin, our mouths stuffed with bread, the couple made it back to their table and just stared at it. Henry noticed the wide-eyed look of horror on my face as I tried silently to turn his attention to the crab claw sticking out of the top of his shirt. He adjusted it quickly.

We tried hard not to look in their direction as they looked around and wondered what had happened to their dinners. We tried hard not to laugh as they called the waiter over to ask where their dinners were. We tried hard not to choke on the remaining clumps of chewed garlic bread in our mouths when the waiter started yelling at the busboy. We must have looked odd holding our arms across our chests, staring at the salt shakers, our shoulders heaving in silent hysteria.

It all ended well for the couple. They made up and were holding hands as they were given fresh new platters of seafood; meanwhile, we sat there waiting in great discomfort for our bill in our butter-stained clothing.

Whether God punished me for eating other people's food or for not sticking to my diet, I will never know. But the next time Henry, Artie, and John decide to go out for dinner, I'll wait in the car.

## SURVIVAL HINTS

1. Always try to eat well-balanced and healthy meals; it'll help you avoid the temptation to steal other people's dinners.
2. If you are on a road trip with crazy friends, try to plan ahead and bring healthy snacks along in the car to avoid embarrassing adventures with food.

# Hershey:
# Or Dieting Isn't Sane

*Ray Zardetto*

GOING CRAZY TRYING to lose weight? There's a simple reason why: Sanity and dieting do not go together.

If you accept the simple premise that dieting is an act of insanity in America, you have a good chance of staying sane. If you don't think it's an act of insanity to try cutting calories in this day and age, stop for a moment and understand what you are up against.

Have you ever visited the Hershey's Chocolate Factory in Hershey, Pennsylvania? On its chocolate-making tour, Hershey boasts that it turns out more than 70 million chocolate kisses *every day*. According to Hershey's labeling, nine of those innocent-looking little bite-sized kisses contain 230 calories. That's more than twenty-five calories per kiss. Think about that.

That means Hershey lets loose in the marketplace more than 1,700,000,000 calories *every day* in chocolate kisses! Add to that the dozens of other chocolate bars and candies Hershey makes, then multiply that by the dozens of other chocolate and candy makers all over the world and you're talking calorie numbers that have to be measured in light years. And that's just candy!

On top of that, you've got restaurants trying to outdo each other by offering larger and larger portions of food until they have to serve them by way of steam shovels instead of waiters. You've got fast-food restaurants on every highway in every town offering basic meals with calorie counts that would choke African elephants. And don't forget the fillers, additives, and sugars that seem to be added to everything from fruit juice to filet mignon.

Is it any wonder a dieter can go crazy?

Some perspective here might also help you hold on to your sanity.

Americans haven't collectively figured out effective ways to diet because we haven't been at it long enough. The idea of dieting is a relatively new phenomenon—mainly because having so many fat people in America is also a pretty new phenomenon.

Remaining thin was a lot easier for those who came before us. Our forefathers and foremothers lived in an agrarian society. The only food they saw was what they grew or churned out themselves (literally). If the harvest didn't work out for a particular year, then bark chips and grass were the "special du jour." Who's going to order second helpings with cuisine like that?

Your great-great-great ancestors didn't need fad diets or programs. Can you imagine Colonial Weight Watchers? "Huzzah to Jedidiah for he hath lost four pounds this fortnight!" "And woe to you, Ezekiel— thou needest deny thyself mutton and pudding lest thy horse be no longer able to support thee!"

I'm not excusing fat people. Everyone who needs to lose weight, as I do, should lose weight. There are many good reasons to do it—and remembering these reasons can help you keep a firm grasp on your sanity.

Being overweight can lead to all kinds of physical problems—especially as you grow older. Some experts say that obesity can lead to psychological problems as well, but I won't be convinced of that until I see a fat serial killer.

In addition, the calorie-challenged among us have limited career opportunities. You don't see fat astronauts, chimney sweeps, limbo dancers, ballerinas, submarine officers, or glider pilots, do you? On the other hand, staying fat is okay if you aspire to be a professional cannon-baller in the neighborhood swimming pool or you plan on making a living by selling shade at the beach.

How do you know whether you should lose weight?

Not everyone who thinks he or she needs to lose weight should. I have met many people, mostly women, who are as thin as a rail but say they have to drop another five or ten pounds. I look at them and wonder how they can lose any more weight without cutting off a limb.

On the other hand, if you are what you eat, some people look as if they have been nibbling on a 747 Airbus for too long. I suspect that if the post office has proposed giving you your own ZIP code, or you are developing your own gravitational pull, then a few months at the salad bar are probably in order.

Your best bet would be to consult your physician before you start. He or she will know what is best for you. If you don't have a physician, I suggest you get one before you start dieting. In fact, I strongly suggest you go to a fat physician. He or she will probably go easier on you.

Two important things before you start: First, set a realistic goal. Don't go by the nutrition and weight guides set by the Food and Drug Administration

(FDA). You ever see those? They seem appropriate for greyhounds, not humans. These charts are not realistic and the only explanation is that they were created by using prisoners on hunger strikes as benchmarks.

Second, I strongly suggest that you go out and buy some pants that are two or three sizes larger than your current waist size. About a week into your diet, begin to wear these new pants. You will feel as if you have accomplished a lot.

Don't diet alone. Misery loves company. Select a companion dieter with whom you can commiserate and compete as you lose weight.

There are two ways to approach the selection process. First, if you plan to be disciplined and follow through on your diet regimen, then you should pick as a companion someone you dislike. That way, when you achieve your goals, you can double your satisfaction if your companion fails.

On the other hand, if you don't think you will stay the course, pick a good friend as a dieting companion. That way, if he or she succeeds and you don't, you won't feel so bad.

It goes without saying that this companion should weigh more—a lot more—than you do.

Here is an idea that is extremely effective—but it requires you to develop your self-denial (I'm assuming you don't already practice self-denial—otherwise you wouldn't need to diet).

Think of something you don't have but you *really, really* want—the more expensive the better! Something embarrassingly expensive as a manifest goal can provide you a rock of sanity during the crazy drudgery of daily dieting.

When you reach your weight-loss goal, make sure you buy whatever it is you've set your heart on. Again, the more expensive the prize the better—it will leave you with less money for food and a better chance of keeping the weight off.

## SURVIVAL HINTS

1. Set realistic goals for your diet so that you won't be frustrated because they are impossible to achieve.
2. Diet with a buddy to keep you motivated and to take away the monotony. Misery loves company!
3. Pick a reward and be sure to get it for yourself when you hit your goal. Bribery works well, and it'll help you stay motivated.

# When You're on a Brand-Name Diet

# Sanity Quiz

You have started the latest craze dieting plan that guarantees rapid weight loss in record time. However, you never read the fine print and this diet is making you fatter than you were to begin with.

Do you

A. hunt down the developer and give him a piece of your mind
B. write a press release describing the bad effects of this plan
C. suck it up and try something else
D. all of the above

If you answered yes to any of these questions, read on and find out how our contributors made some famous diet plans work for them—their advice is solid and their stories will make you chuckle.

# My Date with Jenny Craig

*Dennis Purdy*

DIETING HAS NEVER BEEN my thing. I never really had to worry about it, but in 1995 I found myself in my forties, "suddenly" thirty pounds overweight and making myself all kinds of shallow promises—the kinds many of us make to ourselves, I suppose—to start doing something about it . . . *sometime soon.*

My "sometime soon" came on September 5, 1995, at 11:55 a.m. I remember the exact time because it was five minutes before my son's kindergarten class let out and the exact moment that Kathy walked into my life. Like me and a handful of other parents milling around outside the classroom door, she was waiting to pick up her daughter from the first day of school.

I had been divorced for several years and Kathy, who wasn't wearing a ring, intrigued me from the moment I first set eyes on her outside that kindergarten class. During our small talk, I learned that she worked as a Jenny Craig weight loss consultant. *"Great,"* I told myself. *"I have finally met someone I'm interested in and it has to be a weight loss professional who can obviously see that I'm lousy at watching what I eat."*

After collecting our kids, we walked to the parking lot and carried on our conversation for another ten minutes or so. By the time Kathy left that day, not only was I smitten, I was resolved to lose weight—and Kathy was going to be my Jenny Craig weight loss consultant, even though she didn't yet know it.

During the next two weeks, I went to the school every day, morning and noon, in hopes of seeing Kathy again, but I didn't. I also went cold turkey on my daily ration of six to ten cans of Mountain Dew, several Kit Kat bars, and at least one pack of Twinkies. I wanted to get a jump start on the diet program I knew I'd be undertaking but had not yet officially signed up for. I started getting the sweats and the jitters, unsure whether it was from anxiety over failing to run into Kathy again or because my body was going through severe sugar withdrawal from the one-hundred or so ounces of sugar-laced junk foods that I was no longer putting into my body every day.

Failing to run into Kathy again, I decided to go to Plan B. I went through the phone book and called every Jenny Craig Weight Loss Centre in the book trying to locate the one where the woman I knew only as "Kathy" worked. Finally, the last one I called was the right one and the manager was quite happy to assign Kathy as my weight loss consultant because we already "knew" each other.

I was quite nervous when I walked into the Jenny Craig Weight Loss Centre for my first appointment. I was also proud of myself because in the two weeks since I'd met Kathy, I'd succeeded in losing nine pounds. Whether she could see the difference or not, I could, and it felt good.

Since it was my initial visit, I had to fill out about six hundred forms, including one that asked the question, "Why do you want to lose weight?" Hmm. I was in a quandary. Should I give the real answer—"I fell in love at first sight with one of your weight loss consultants and this is the only way I'm going to see her again"—or should I write something else? I decided to put down something else because I'm basically a chicken at heart when it comes to romance: "I want to live a long and healthy life and make sure my two kids grow to adulthood and can make a living on their own without having to go live with their selfish witch of a mother, who abandoned us all two years ago." That seemed like a safe, politically correct answer.

Once I had filled out the six hundred forms, Kathy had me pose for a Polaroid "before" picture, which was then promptly placed on the bulletin board for all of the county's 400,000 citizens to see. Geez, those nine pounds I had lost sure didn't seem to show up. Well, I figured, it must be the difference between Polaroid pictures and regular pictures. (I would learn later that it's entirely normal for people who are dieting to do a lot of this kind of absurd rationalizing.) My first session with Kathy was perfunctory. The insanity of my first two weeks of dieting was taking its toll. "What's wrong with her?" I thought. "Can't she tell I'm madly in love with her and would happily chop off both feet in order to lose enough weight to please her?" No, probably not. Why, I wondered, can't women ever sense the good things about a man? Are they so focused on weight loss when they're in a weight loss establishment that they can't see the bigger picture?

I left the Jenny Craig Weight Loss Centre that day with enough dieting papers to choke a horse and about twelve hundred dollars worth of food and videos; I was hoping—but not sure—that Kathy would get some kind of commission from my purchases. I was willing to buy more, but they were out of stock for about nine or ten of their videos.

I drove home in silence except for the two little guys on my shoulders. You know, the slender one dressed all in white who looks like Pat Boone and whispers encouragement ("You can do it! You can lose the weight!") and the fat one, dressed all in red, chomping on a Twinkie, guzzling a Mountain Dew, screaming in a perfect Sam Kinison imitation, "Fat chance, fat boy! It'll never work! Your motivation is all wrong. You love the sweets too much and she doesn't even know you exist!"

When I arrived home, I set all the food, videos, and horse-choking papers on the kitchen counter in a big pile. I just wanted to gaze upon my twelve hundred dollars worth of weight-loss insanity one more time before I put the food in the freezer, the videos on the top shelf of a closet I never used, and the papers in the garbage can. Then I began to feel a bit foolish about what I had done. Maybe the miniature Sam Kinison on my shoulder was right. This will never work. My motivation for losing weight *was* all wrong. And what was this stuff about only eighteen hundred calories a day? I *was* supposed to stay alive while I was dieting, wasn't I?

Before actually undertaking the ritual of disposing of my insanity's evidence, I noticed the little shirt-pocket-sized food log in which I was supposed to write down every morsel and every drop that passed my lips and entered my belly. Great. Not only had I volunteered to be tortured—and had paid for the pleasure (agony) of it—they even expected me to document it! Strange. Kathy hadn't seemed so sadistic when I first met her.

Sam Kinison was right. This wasn't going to work. I had only been on my diet for twenty-two minutes and thirty-eight seconds and I was already depressed. "This isn't right," I thought. "The depression over failure to lose weight isn't supposed to come until later, like, at least eight or ten hours. Right?"

I left all the Jenny Craig paraphernalia sitting on the kitchen counter in the afternoon sun in one giant compost pile that I was hoping would somehow spontaneously combust and, with a jittery hand, took out a can of Mountain Dew from the refrigerator and popped the top. I downed the can of soda without stopping to take a breath.

As I continued to stare at my expensive compost pile, I began to be aware of the starkly contrasting emotions that were running through me. Part of me felt better after having consumed the can of Mountain Dew in what surely must have been world record time, yet part of me felt bad for having done so. Geez, does everyone who diets become so conflicted? Do Pat

Boone and Sam Kinison pay personal visits to everyone who diets?

I immediately came to two conclusions. First, the miracle of spontaneous combustion wasn't about to visit my house that day, so I might as well come up with a workable solution for making the most of the compost pile. Second, I should undertake some serious and mature self-assessment about this dieting thing I had insanely agreed to, and if I drank another Mountain Dew while sitting in my recliner as I self-assessed with Pat and Sam during Monday Night Football, it wouldn't really hurt. (There's that dieter's rationalization thing again.)

Midway through the first quarter—and a second Mountain Dew—I realized that losing weight in an effort to become more attractive to the opposite sex wasn't an entirely wrong motive. If that's the motivation I needed to do the right thing for my health, then so be it. At least I was getting it done. I eventually kicked Sam out and let Pat move in, and I lost thirty-seven pounds in about three months on the Jenny Craig Weight Loss program.

Yes, my initial motivation was to meet Kathy and the actual goal of weight loss was secondary. But I still lost the weight. So, the encouragement I offer about staying sane while dieting is to find something so important to *you* that it will be worth going through the jitters and shakes of sugar withdrawal, the derogatory screaming of your own Sam Kinison, and the painstaking effort of becoming a more mature, healthy person.

And Kathy? Ten years later, she is my best friend and sweetheart, and I thank God that in 1995, I was thirty-seven pounds overweight.

Dennis Purdy is the author of *The Illustrated Guide to Texas Hold'em: Making Winners Out of Beginners and Advanced Players* (Sourcebooks, 2005); *The Team-by-Team Encyclopedia of Baseball* (Workman, 2006); and *The Ultimate Baseball Trivia Book* (Workman, 2006).

# Doing Atkins
# the Feldman Way

*Harvey Feldman*

WE HAD JUST RETURNED home from a late January
vacation. This restful eating orgy followed the obliga-
tory bingeing and gorging between Thanksgiving and
New Year's. Sitting down to dinner, my wife announced, "*I've* put on a few pounds lately. *We* have to
go on a diet." "Okay," I said, thinking that while I was
still relatively thin (by *my* standards), a diet might be
fun. After all, since we were married (more than thirty
years ago) I had allowed myself to gain a measly one
pound a year (okay, a pound and a quarter), but I car-

ried most of the extra weight around my middle where no one could see it (right!).

The diet of choice was Atkins, selected by my wife because she thought the basic tenets agreed to some extent with my own philosophy of eating and exercising (a lot of good it had done me) and because recent publicity suggested that it might actually work. I had never been on a real diet before; indeed, I had always reveled in my after-dinner snacks of ice cream, chocolate, and more chocolate. So this foray into Atkins represented quite a change from my customary habits.

After reading every book by and about Atkins, we were ready to begin. We dutifully followed the "induction" phase, which eliminates virtually all carbohydrates. The recommended period for this phase is two weeks, but because I'm compulsive, I stayed with it for four. I figured that if two weeks is good, four must be better! My wife, however, was eager to reintroduce vegetables into her diet, so she jumped ahead to the "maintenance" phase after the requisite two weeks.

One of the objectives of eating fewer carbs and more fat is to achieve ketosis, a state in which your body is retrained to burn fat. Among the unfortunate side effects is severe bad breath, which now takes on the odor of rotting garbage. Unpleasant, yes, and definitely not an appetite stimulant!

Believe it or not, I actually enjoyed eliminating empty carbohydrates from my diet, and I was pleased to find that the usual humongous cheese omelet I had for breakfast was totally acceptable. And I was happy to eat all the fish, meat, cheese, and salad I could ingest during the day. Before long, I was able to add "allowable" snacks, such as nuts and an occasional "no sugar" chocolate bar. Of course, I missed bread, pasta, French fries, and cookies, but seeing the pounds drop away every few days provided enough positive reinforcement to stay with it.

My wife, in the meantime, was experiencing "fruit withdrawal" and was anticipating a new phase. To make a long story a bit shorter, at the end of four months I had lost twenty-four pounds (my goal was twenty), and my wife had lost twenty-four ounces. She was not a happy camper. I have followed the Atkins approach for about two years now, and kept the weight off (except for brief fluctuations of no more than five pounds). During the same two years, my wife tried various diets, including the Zone, the South Beach, and the Mediterranean. How much additional weight has she lost? She's not telling! But if you add up all the weight she says she's lost over the years, I'm sure it equals a small SUV.

From my experience and observation, I can recommend Atkins for men who seriously want to lose weight, have more energy, eliminate the afternoon "drowsies," and maybe reduce their cholesterol (I checked mine before and during the diet, and my cholesterol and triglyceride levels are significantly lower than they were before I started my diet), or even improve their overall health. For some inexplicable reason, Atkins seems to be more effective for men than for women.

But for any diet to work you need to make exercise a regular part of your life (you probably should even if you're not on a diet). A nice thing about Atkins is that once you've reached your goal, occasional dietary transgressions (yes, even pizza, tacos, and Häagen-Dazs) won't put permanent pounds back on if you go back to the "induction" phase for a few days immediately afterwards. Doubling up your exercise routine for a week or so couldn't hurt, either!

Another positive result of losing weight and keeping it off: I wanted to reward myself for achieving my goal, and I celebrated with a good cigar. I enjoyed it so much that cigars have become a regular treat for me! And there is another benefit: I've been able to wear clothes that haven't fit me for the past ten years (yes, I still have clothes from thirty years ago, when I was first married). Being thin (all right, "thinner") definitely has its rewards.

I'm so glad that *we* had to start dieting when *we* did, and while my wife continues to bounce from diet to diet, I'll never have to go on a "diet" again! I don't think of it as a "diet" anymore, but rather as a lifestyle change, something that I can continue for as long as I want. It was a challenge, it was fun, and the final result (for me, anyway) made it all worthwhile.

Oh, one last note. I'm now able to indulge my chocolate craving with small quantities of "real" chocolate (bittersweet dark only) whenever I feel the urge, without guilt and without gaining weight. And I've recently discovered the most delicious organic dark chocolate laced with chili peppers that I can indulge in whenever the urge strikes. Life is good!

## SURVIVAL HINTS

1. Do your research before starting a diet to be sure you want to undertake it. Knowing what's involved will help you make the right choice for you.
2. Once you pick a diet, commit to sticking to it for at least four to six weeks, long enough to see whether it's working for you.
3. Don't be too hard on yourself if the diet you have chosen is not right for you. Not every diet works for every dieter. If the pounds don't start to disappear, try a different approach.

4.  Don't give up on losing weight. Be patient. Remember, if you can make a lifestyle change that helps you shed those pounds, you'll never have to diet again!

5.  Exercise is critical. Try to find at least twenty minutes a day for some type of workout (e.g., calisthenics, isometrics, jumping rope, weights, Tai Bo) and you'll create a powerful synergy for super-charging your diet.

# Watch Out for
# Weight Watchers

*Arline Simpson*

*Dieting per the thesaurus: Watch your weight; watch your waistline; watch what you eat; cut down; starve yourself; reduce.*

SO THERE I WAS, forty years old, the mother of three children, and a survivor of breast cancer, a mastectomy, a hysterectomy, and twenty-five radiation treatments, all of which had left me weighing in at 115 pounds. But now I was up to 140 pounds and gaining.

So off I went to Weight Watchers—scared to death and frustrated.

I had given up eating sweets.

I had given up drinking wine.

I ate lots of fruit and vegetables.

But I was still gaining weight.

When I got there, I signed in, gave them my personal data—height, weight, age—they weighed me, gave me a booklet, and sent me into the room where a woman was standing in front of a microphone. She was talking about food.

Behind her was a chart showing all the things one should eat, and exactly how much.

Back in those days, there were no points, no ready-prepared brand-name meals, just calories to count.

The women sitting in folding chairs around me were at least twenty-five to seventy-five pounds heavier than I was, but that didn't make me feel any better about my protruding backside, thighs, and stomach.

Even though I admitted to myself that I was better dressed and made up than they were, and I appeared to have at least some control over myself compared to my compatriots, I still couldn't button my slacks. And that awful tightness around my thighs was uncomfortable.

Even though my husband thought I looked great, my sister was much heavier than I was, and my coworkers always complimented me on my appearance, I was still unhappy. Those bulges just wouldn't go away. They plagued me night and day. I measured myself with a tape measure every week, and I weighed myself daily. I purchased a calorie counter book and diary, and I tried to write down every morsel of food I ingested. But despite all that effort, there I was, at Weight Watchers, with all those dowdy women.

The lecture began. It sounded like this:

Ladies and gentlemen, I am here to help you reach your goals. You have done nothing wrong by choice, but you do not know how to balance your intake.

All you need to do is understand how to control and balance your food intake so that you achieve the optimum nourishment and do not gain weight.

She proceeded to tell us which foods contain which vitamins and minerals, how many calories each morsel contained, and how to weigh and measure our intake.

This was fact, so I listened, but then she began to speak about ways to avoid bingeing.

She suggested that we wear rubber gloves when preparing food. Why? Because no one wants to eat food that tastes like a rubber glove.

She even had all the equipment we'd need to get started, including small scales for weighing our food, measuring cups, spoons, and utensils. She also recommended different brands of food that contained the right types and numbers of calories.

Then it was our turn to tell her about our poor eating habits. It was like confession. These women told scary stories: They got up in the middle of the night and ate candy and cake; they hid cookies from their children and husbands; and they binged on pizza and beer. They overdosed on chocolate, junk food, and McDonalds' burgers; Twinkies were big, but Mallomars were the favorite. Ice cream was another huge pitfall. When they realized what this junk was doing, they resorted to buttered popcorn by the gallon.

Laxatives became a big issue, and so did diuretics. Take some, lose some, and then resume your old habits.

I became frightened by their stories. And even though my ignorance was not as severe as that of the gathered confessors, I, too, had gained too much weight and was necessarily there with the rest of them.

I started the diet. After three weeks, I had lost only two pounds, not the two pounds a week it was suggested I could lose.

After two months at Weight Watchers, I got with the program, followed the diet faithfully, and ultimately lost fifteen pounds. I was definitely the better for it.

But I don't think the diet helped me nearly as much as the stories I listened to every week at the meetings. Those women scared me! I didn't know that people actually hid food in their night tables, behind couches and closets, in canisters, and anywhere else they could think of.

And you never know how you'll end up using what you learn at those meetings. I adopted some of these same strategies after my husband underwent quintuple bypass surgery and was not supposed to sneak in extra treats, especially sweets and high-fat snacks. So now, not only am I careful what I cook for him but I also hide my stash of chocolate in some of the same creative hiding places revealed to me so long ago at my early Weight Watchers meetings. Those women may have scared me, but they also taught me some useful things; for example, sometimes a little deception is the way to go. As long as my husband doesn't attend Weight Watchers meetings, my secret stash— and his diet—will be safe!

# 3

# When You Cheat
# on Your Diet

### *A Good Diet Gone Bad*
Joyce Romano

### *Confessions of a Fat Teenager*
Mia Bennay

### *Diary of a Cheater*
Lara Ledfeld

# Sanity Quiz

You are waiting for the bus while standing in front of your favorite bakery. The bus should arrive any minute, but the baker places your favorite double-chocolate layer cake in the front window and now you have to make a choice.

Do you

A. take your chances on missing the bus and sprint into the bakery
B. run in and ask for just a small slice
C. press a twenty on the window and have the baker bring you out a piece
D. stick to your guns and wait patiently for the bus

If you answered yes to A, B, or C, then you're ready to find out how our writers went astray. You'll see yourself in some of them, and you'll have a good laugh at the same time. After all, misery does love company.

# A Good Diet Gone Bad

*Joyce Romano*

RACHEL, WHO HAD JUST GONE on a strict diet two
weeks earlier, was dangerously late for her flight
home. As she ran to catch the plane, she was also
aware that she was absolutely famished. Having no
time to seek out a low-cal, low-carb snack for her diet
du jour, she sought out something quick to put in her
stomach. She hated cheating on a new diet, but she
absolutely had to eat something.

She ran into the newsstand near her boarding gate
and spent too many precious moments agonizing over
the nutritional value of a Kit Kat as opposed to a
Snickers bar. "Oh, thank goodness, no one on my diet
team is watching," she thought.

The Kit Kat won.

So a sweaty and stressed Rachel, the Kit Kat, and today's paper boarded the flight with three seconds to spare. While she stuffed the items into her briefcase, she pushed down the aisle to find her seat—19C, a window seat. She was now hoping that she would have the whole row of seats to herself as a consolation for the hungry, grumpy, and stressed condition she had found herself in.

More irritation. She would not be sitting alone. She even had to climb over a very fat man in the aisle seat who was already snoring away in dreamland. "Well," she thought, "at least the center seat is free. And hopefully Fat Albert here will sleep the whole flight and not want to chat."

Rachel put her briefcase on the seat, pulled out her paper, and started reading. But soon hunger got the better of her, and she grabbed the Kit Kat bar, snapped off a section, and savored the sweet guilty pleasure of the chocolate flavor for a moment, then went back to her newspaper.

Sensing movement next to her, Rachel concentrated more deeply on the article she was reading so that she wouldn't encourage conversation from the waking man. Out of the corner of her eye, she saw him lean over, grab her Kit Kat bar from the middle seat, snap off a section, and eat it. Rachel was flabbergasted! What nerve! She wasn't sure whether she should say something and risk a long, tense flight, or whether she should just let it go. Instead, Rachel grabbed the Kit Kat bar and broke off another section; after all, what better way to give a subtle hint: "Hands off my candy, mister!"

Within minutes, she saw the man grab the remaining section of the candy bar and pop it in his mouth. But this was an outrage!

Rachel sat silently fuming about this turn of events on an already irritating day. But because his boldness was so intimidating, she said nothing. For the rest of the flight, no words were exchanged between the two warring candy eaters.

After the flight, Rachel raced to the carousel to pick up her baggage. She saw the fat man standing there and started an internal conversation with herself about all the clever and biting things she could have said to him about his rude behavior. But the man's bags arrived before hers and he headed off for the coffee shop. She felt disgusted with herself for being so timid and feeling like a victim.

A few minutes later, she finally spotted her bag, grabbed it from the carousel, and instead of heading for the exit, changed direction and entered the coffee shop. She intended to confront the man.

She saw him sitting at the counter with a cup of coffee and a donut. Without a word, Rachel seized the donut and stuffed the whole thing into her mouth like a crazed caveman. Then she picked up his cup of coffee, took a long swig, and slammed it back down on the counter. He was staring at her with his mouth open as he watched her wipe her wet coffee lips across her suit sleeve. Laughing like a demon and covered in crumbs, Rachel ran out of the shop. She felt vindicated.

Some moments later in the taxicab, Rachel, still seething, was telling her driver the Kit Kat story, blaming the audacious fat man for forcing her to eat a donut and completely blow her diet. Then, as she was rummaging around in her briefcase for her wallet to pay the driver, she saw something shocking . . . a Kit Kat bar.

I suppose that in the future, Rachel, having learned her lesson the hard and embarrassing way, will either take the airlines' advice and make sure that her snack, like her checked baggage, is truly her own, or else risk once again becoming the madly munching maniac who let a good diet go bad.

## SURVIVAL HINTS

1. Always try to eat well-balanced and regularly timed meals to avoid snacking on candy.

2. If you must have a snack and are confronted only with convenience store items such as candy and pretzels, reach for the pretzels first. They contain less fat and fewer calories, and they won't give you a sugar slump.

3. If you are either starving or bingeing on sugar, you may not be totally rational, so try to avoid both!

# Confessions of a Fat Teenager

*Mia Bennay*

I WAS A FAT KID. Roly-poly. Rather rotund. A chu-bette. I had to buy chubby sizes in a whole different department of the kids' clothing store, and it was *soooo* embarrassing. Not only that, but the other kids called me names. "Blimp" was the politest of the bunch. It was awful.

When I hit the teen years, I decided that enough was enough. I was going to change things and that was that. So I went on a major diet for the first and only time in my life.

I used a multipronged plan of attack. Rather than snacking all day long, which was what I'd done for most of my life, I ate only at mealtimes. This had to reduce my intake of calories by about 200 percent, and that alone made a big difference.

Next, I decided to cut back on my portions. Instead of eating a full helping, I ate only half. These two items drastically cut my intake of food, calories, fat, and bulk.

Then I started eliminating fat, especially saturated fat, from everything I ate. I began reading the labels of all the foods in the house. I stopped ingesting mountains of French fries and other greasy foods, all big offenders.

Finally, I cut out desserts until I was confident that my weight was dropping as I'd hoped it would. I decided that when I had lost thirty pounds, I'd revisit the dessert question.

If I got hungry, I drank water or unsweetened beverages. If I was really starving, I ate celery.

And what happened was miraculous. After six months, I'd dropped all the excess weight, and I looked more like the pictures of the girls in the magazines I read each month—I'd *done* it!

About twenty-five years ago, I decided to join a gym, and then I not only weighed in at my goal, but also my body became firmer and stronger—an added bonus. Even my doctor asked what I was doing to myself because my body was so different from the way it was previously at annual visits. I told him, and he was pleased. Not only that, but all my test results were perfect.

Now, almost forty years after that chubby little teenager went on that first and only diet, I am still that same petite person I'd become way back in high school. It's not that hard once you make up your mind.

## SURVIVAL HINTS

1. Cut out all between-meal snacks to cut out extra calories. You might actually cut your intake in half using this simple technique.
2. Try leaving half your portion of each normal serving of food. This will cut your calories in half again.
3. Avoid saturated fats, which put on the pounds fast.
4. Go to the gym at least three times a week. This will help speed up your metabolism and help you burn fat and calories in record time; and the exercise will give you extra energy, too, which, in turn, will help you become more active naturally!

# Diary of a Cheater

*Lara Ledfeld*

"What's just one pastry?" I said to myself. That was on top of the other fifty "just ones" I had eaten over the course of this diet. I was a cheater, a fully fledged dieting adulterer. I would sneak out late at night just to meet my true love—food. I would tell myself this was okay because no one else knew what I was doing. But I was cheating only myself. I would eat only at darkened restaurants, where I was unrecognizable. I would make secret calls from my cell phone and book myself at some of the finest restaurants in town so that no one else saw them on the home bill. I would pay for everything in cash so that the meals could not be traced to my credit card. I was as careful as any philanderer ever was.

That's because I was "The Mad Dieter." This insanity had overcome me like the plague. And now it wasn't about me and my weight anymore—it had become a game, a veritable obsession. It was like an overwhelming affair. My mind had been working overtime for so long about what I could and couldn't eat that I finally just gave in to it. Now I was insane, insane over food, totally and completely mad about it.

I claimed to be on a diet, but I indulged in some of the finest foods available. While my family sat at home and suffered with my "diet menu," I was sneaking around, stuffing my face elsewhere, enjoying extracurricular meals and snacks on all sides. I literally had my cake and ate it, too. I was on a path of self-destruction, and sooner or later I would be caught, as most cheaters are. I could not justify the reasons for my odd behavior other than as a cry for help. Maybe I really wanted to get caught.

As my weight increased, so did my family's suspicions. I knew something had to be done—I was out of control. My double life of dieting had caused me to gain forty additional pounds. One day, while I feasted in a local restaurant, I was confronted by my entire family. They had secretly followed me. I was caught full-fisted: A large roll in one hand and a fork full of pie in the other. And that was the day I confessed. I told my family everything, everything I had done, purchased, and ultimately eaten. I finally came clean about my secret love affair with food, and I was ready to accept their scorn and the consequences of my lies.

Thankfully, that confession set me free! My family understood and forgave my deceptions. They were relieved that the real cause of my weight gain was from a lack of self-discipline and determination rather than a serious health problem. My cheating days were over, and now not only did I lose those extra pounds but I could look people in the eye, a cheater no more!

## SURVIVAL HINTS

1. Be honest with yourself when you're trying to diet. Cheating won't help you lose weight.
2. If you're having a hard time sticking to your diet, ask for help from someone who's been successful at dieting. If that doesn't work, consider seeing a nutrition counselor or going to one of the diet programs where motivation and regular weigh-ins might keep you on the straight and narrow!

**4**

# When You Design
# Your Own Diet

*The Half and Double Diet*
Winston Habrick

*Scone-Free Sanity*
Melissa Wadsworth

*The Potato-Chip Diet*
Evelyn M. Fazio

*The Snapping Diet*
Rusty Fellini

*The No-Diet Diet*
Samantha Hearns

# Sanity Quiz

You are on a diet and everything seems to be going well. All of a sudden you realize you are slowly gaining back all of the weight you fought so hard to lose.

Do you

A. pay closer attention to what you're eating
B. dismiss the gain as a freak happening
C. assure yourself that you lost it once, so the second time around will not be a problem
D. all of the above

If you answered yes to any of these questions, you need to read on. If you're winging it on your own brand of diet and it's not working, check out how these folks made their plans work for them. You'll find some great and original ideas that you can build into your own plan.

# The Half and Double Diet

*Winston Habrick*

I ALWAYS USED TO WALK to work because I didn't want to own a car. But then I started getting rides from one of my staff members. We worked together and were good friends, so it was fun to chat and laugh on the brief ride home.

But I also started to gain weight. And it wasn't just that. We went out to lunch a few times a week to escape the insanity at our company after the less-than-pleasant change in management had brought with it crazy and counterproductive ways of doing things. The result was that now I was eating more and walking less. Not a good combination.

Not only that, but I was also cooking a lot more than ever, and eating a lot, too. I was having a wonderful time, but my waistline was hanging over my belt a little too much.

Finally I decided that I was enjoying too much of a good thing, so I came up with my very own diet, and it's worked well for me for many years. In fact, as a result of this plan, I now weigh the same as I did when I graduated from high school, and I'm in my sixties.

It's called the "Half and Double Diet." And here's how it works.

First, you halve all your portions. And I mean *all* of them. If you normally eat two eggs for breakfast, now you have one. If you normally eat two cheeseburgers for lunch, now eat one. If you normally eat a big steak for dinner, eat only half. If you are used to eating two pieces of bread with your meal, eat just one. The same applies to drinks—other than water.

Second, double your activity. If you always take the elevator up two flights, get out and walk up one flight. If you normally park in front of the door to your office, park halfway across the lot. If you vacuum only one room a day, now vacuum two. If you are sedentary, get up and go for a walk for five minutes to begin with, then after a few weeks increase your walk to ten minutes.

I started out walking a mile each day, and now I'm up to four. I have lost weight, I am never out of breath, and my legs are as strong as tree trunks. Not only that, but I never get colds, the flu, or anything else.

So if you've put on a few pounds over the winter, or if you've enjoyed a little too much of a good thing, try my Half and Double Diet plan. Before you know it, you'll be in better shape than ever and the envy of all your friends!

# Scone-Free Sanity

*Melissa Wadsworth*

ONE DAY I REALIZED that I was wearing middle age. And it wasn't pretty. There it was on my thighs, hips, waist, and arms. There was a middling roundness in my face.

Perhaps it was falling in love in Seattle, the coffee capital of America, that had done me in. Every cup of rich brew screamed for a scone—blueberry, orange-cinnamon, fruit-and-nut. Honey-soaked bran muffins beckoned from their glass cases, enticing partners in crime. My senses were as open to each new taste sensation as they were to all the new experiences of touch, smell, sight, and sound that I was enjoying romantically. What was not to love?

A sense of moderation had no place in this scenario. There were no "no's" in my love vocabulary. I indulged, wallowed in the power of the affirmative: "Yes, I want this," "Yes, I would like that," "Yes, more please." Yet, as liberating, as fully sensual as it was (emotionally and appetite-wise), I slowly began to see the consequences of a cup that so fully runneth over. Indeed, the consequences appeared fully formed: Donut-shaped rings of fat rimmed my upper thighs, dimpled batter accessorized my waistline, and my upper arms rounded out as stoutly as a certain dough-boy's. It wasn't that I didn't exercise, I did. I had just stopped exercising common sense.

This reality (no longer softly screened by new love) abruptly ended my liberation from moderation. A diet loomed upon the horizon, unwelcome yet inevitable. Not even love could disguise the fact that I was seeing my mother's form in the mirror looking back at me kindly and softly, yet she was clearly disapproving.

Yet, I had a dilemma. What form of denial could I accept as a forty-something dieter who has been there and done that? I had tried the original Atkins diet in the 1970s during the first low-carb fad, but it held little allure for me now (okay, so I hated it). My grown-sensitive-over-the-years digestion would not tolerate a grapefruit diet, nor any other eat-only-one-kind-of-food prescription. A low-fat regime faired just as poorly because it could not stand up to my mature knowledge about the health benefits of good oils and unsaturated fats. Before I reached the age of thirty I had experienced the craziness of dieting in nearly every form offered: peel-a-pound soup, liquid diets, compulsive calorie counting. I knew well the end to those circuitous roads.

There was but one solution: I needed to remove the original offender—sugar and flour. I had to admit it. I can't withstand the power of a little sugar. One bite one day and the next I find myself sniffing out the next sweet treat, my fix, as naturally as a squirrel nosing through a favorite nut cache. So the offender had to go completely. Much easier, I reasoned, to eradicate the source of trouble than to scale it back. Sugar has devious ways of disguising its size, its impact, of appearing like a small vice, a friendly companion. Better not to invite it along at all. Also, as lovely as its manifestations could be, white flour offered no real nutritional value, so it made sense to relinquish its hold, too.

The first day was the hardest. By mid-afternoon, my sugar-craving body wondered where its treat was. It reminded me of the backwoods folktale home remedy for tapeworms shared by my seventh grade science teacher (more legend than truth): Each hour, for eight hours, eat a cookie. On the ninth hour, do not.

When the tapeworm appears asking where its cookie is, grab it and pull it out. That vision alone was enough to prevent me from caving in to temptation.

The second and third days presented continued challenges. I warned myself that it was going to be difficult and that this was to be expected. So that I wouldn't be caught off guard when the desire for a little something sweet appeared, I didn't rationalize the itsy-bitsy feeding of the loveable monster. Instead, I would say to myself, "Just as I thought, this is really hard. I must be working in the right direction."

I prepared for the battle with oatmeal and blueberries in the morning. The warm texture and pop of blue color was satisfying and appetite-suppressing for hours. In the beginning, foods such as delectable baked sweet potatoes reminded me of the wonderful natural sweetness available for indulging; they let me convince myself that I really wasn't being deprived; I was only losing my "no-restrictions-in-sight" love fat.

As the weeks and months passed, eating normalcy returned. I relearned the patience of cooking healthy food and of choosing raw treats that weren't all surface sweetness.

I began to taste the natural sweetness of raw pecans, to savor the tropical ripeness of a pineapple. I appreciated again the nutritional bonanza built into a lunch of Miso vegetable soup or mixed green salads graced with pumpkin seeds and a savory olive oil. Dinners of fresh fish with sautéed greens, and the chewy pleasure of wild rice or herbed quinoa eclipsed the memories of buttery scones.

Instead of frozen yogurt in the evenings, teas in a variety of mouth-watering flavors—pear and guava, ginger and liquorice, chamomile and rose hip—appeased my want of something delicious on my tongue.

These days the only thing still clinging to my waist is my human honey, my sweet love, which I never intend to lose.

## SURVIVAL HINTS

1. Choose fresh fruits instead of sugary treats. They'll give you energy and vitamins rather than fat hips, and you'll feel much better without that sugar high and the inevitable sugar plummet that follows.
2. Take your time and keep your expectations realistic, because nobody loses weight overnight. If the weight falls off too fast, you're probably losing only fluids. They will return just as quickly, leaving you very frustrated.
3. Be sure to hug a human rather than a bowl of ice cream—there are fringe benefits, after all!

# The Potato-Chip Diet

*Evelyn M. Fazio*

ONCE I WENT ON a potato-chip diet. Well, actually, the diet followed the potato chips. It all started when a colleague and I began working together over lunch, planning and making decisions while we ate. We worked well together, so we got a lot done, laughed quite a bit, and avoided being stuck in meetings for the rest of the day. The only drawback was that she always brought these amazing sea salt and vinegar potato chips. Every day. No matter what. Blizzards, monsoons, tornadoes—nothing stopped her.

Now I always had, and still have, a weakness for chips, and this particular variety were in their own category of willpower destruction. Kind of like the Holy Grail of chips, as in "Where have these chips been all my life and why didn't someone tell me about them before?" As someone who lived on salad for lunch, and sometimes dinner, too, these chips sang a siren song that threatened to crash me on the rocks of diet-demolition land.

When we were under stress, we ate even more chips. We were trying to make our budget projections, and even though things looked really good, we were both intent not only on attaining our goals but on sur-passing them in hopes of earning a bonus. So we talked, considered, negotiated, approved, rejected, ate lunch, and inhaled a whole big bag a day of those chips. Every day. Five days a week. For months on end.

Soon Chip Heaven became Chip Hell. I started noticing that I didn't have as much room in my waist-bands, and that my clothes didn't look quite right. Time passed. I wasn't really paying attention because I was so consumed with work, and before I knew it: sausage central. I had gained almost twenty pounds!

When I went on vacation to an island in the Caribbean that June, I was determined to break the potato-chip cycle. I tried to eat carefully, and took walks on the beach every day. When I got home, I weighed myself—one pound gone. Okay, it was only a week and only a pound, but it was a beginning. And I had gone a whole week without those chips. I was emboldened to continue life without them.

Next, I stopped eating pasta, bread, potatoes, rice, corn, and all sweets and desserts. I gave up cereal and switched to fruit and yogurt for breakfast, and I took walks every evening after work. After three months of this regimen, not only did my clothes have plenty of extra room but some things were just too big to wear. I was delighted to go get some new, slinky replacements.

After reading that if you exercised before meals, you'd burn off what you ate and speed up the metabolism, I began doing floor exercises every morning before breakfast. My cats thought I was demented. And have you ever tried doing press-ups and cobra stretches with a fifteen-pound cat sitting on your back? It definitely burns some extra calories. The cats got into the act in every way possible: They became leg-lift weights, they smacked my foot as it went up and down, they crouched next to me on the floor and tapped me on the face. Still, I persisted.

Every morning, after the ten minutes of floor exercises and stretches, I used my step machine. It helped burn off some stress, and I was speeding up my metabolism. The cats were entertained, and they watched with amusement as I pumped those steps. Next, I added small weights and additional exercises. And more pounds came off.

But then trouble struck. I injured my back (the problem wasn't exercise-related) and I had to stop *all* exercise for two weeks! I was in a panic. What was I going to do? I felt so much better now that I was getting into shape, and I felt so much less stress after exercising that I was afraid I'd go up in a puff of smoke without it. I didn't see how I'd last, but I survived.

Because I now needed physical therapy for the injury, I learned some wonderful new exercises that not only helped my back but also toned up spots I'd never had success with before. I was thrilled—talk about lemonade from lemons.

Once physical therapy was over, I was hooked on working out. I transferred to the gym at home because I now missed the equipment in the physical therapy workout room, and I managed to replicate the positive effects of using the machines and exercises I'd learned. I added the treadmill and several machines. I had never felt better. Not only that, but with forty-five minutes at the gym three or four times a week, I was able to eat whatever I wanted without gaining an ounce. I stuck to my low-carb life as much as possible, but if I felt like having dessert or an extra treat at a party, it didn't cause too much trouble.

I've lived this way for a long time now, and yes, I even eat the occasional potato chip—but only once in a while. As for my friend with the sea salt and vinegar potato chips, she soon realized that her clothes had gotten much tighter, too, so we decided to end our lunchtime meetings. She brought a bottle of water and some carrot sticks to replace the chips, and I started walking at lunch time and eating a salad at my desk. We still had fun at our meetings, but we ate no more snacks while we worked—it was much safer that way for both of us.

## SURVIVAL HINTS

1. Pay attention to what you eat, and try not to eat while you're doing something else, such as having a meeting or watching television. Awareness keeps you out of trouble!
2. Try to incorporate exercise into your day. It speeds up your metabolism and helps burn off calories.
3. Exercise before meals—you'll burn off what you eat more efficiently. Otherwise, wait at least twenty minutes after meals to exercise so you won't be too full.
4. When beginning an exercise program, do it gradually. Don't start out with too much too soon or you'll be too exhausted to continue.
5. Watch out for potato chips and other junk food snacks—they can fatten you up fast!

# The Snapping Diet

*Rusty Fellini*

I TRIED EVERYTHING. All kinds of diets. Gallons of water, food plans, frozen diets, food deliveries, power bars, liquid diets, everything. Nothing worked. Nada, zilch.

But one day, a friend told me about the snapping diet. I thought he was crazy. What are you supposed to do? Snap your lips all day long while eating as a form of exercise? Snap the refrigerator door shut on your hand? Snap the box of Oreos shut before you eat them all? No, it wasn't any of those, and it turned out to be much easier than any of them.

All you need is a rubber band. Put a rubber band on your wrist. When you think about having a snack, just snap that rubber band. It's kind of like aversion therapy. Soon you won't even want to eat unless you're legitimately hungry. This diet is similar to putting a quarter in a box each time you say a four-letter word if your language is getting too colorful. It helps wake you up to reality and build awareness about what you're doing—and that's really important when you're trying to lose weight. You'll begin to associate the desire for food with the snap, and decide against the snack.

This is really a great diet for people who snack too much. And you know who you are! You are the type of person who grabs a handful of trail mix each time you go past the bowl. Almost as if by magnetic attraction, you turn into a trail mix dust-buster. You aren't really a compulsive eater—but you may just be bored or are not paying attention to what you're shoving into your mouth. Let's call it "auto-stuff."

Auto-stuff especially comes into play when there are a lot of snacks around the office where you work. You know the kind of place I mean—everyone is overweight, they are all on diets, they all complain incessantly about their ever-increasing girth, and yet somewhere there's a table, counter, or empty desk piled with boxes of donuts and coffee cake, bowls of candy, bags of pretzels and chips—all kinds of goodies that will turn you into a parade float or one of those giant parade balloons resembling cartoon characters that can be seen over Fifth Avenue at Thanksgiving. Some of these offices even have schedules: You have to sign up and bring in the snacks during your designated week. This is where auto-stuff runs rampant. If you work in one of these places, avoid signing up. Then they won't let you eat their snacks (just try it— you think that rubber band hurts, but wait until they find an unauthorized muncher in their midst!), and that's a good thing, because it's unlikely that anyone is going to bring in bowls of fresh fruit and vegetables— there'd probably be a mutiny.

But the point of snapping is that if you become aware of what you're eating, you'll start to cut down and lose weight, and it will help you avoid those goodie-laden places at home, at work, or wherever you happen to be. Drink a glass of water each time you snap your wrist, too, and you'll hydrate yourself while you condition yourself.

Another good technique is the food log. No, this is not a log made out of food! It's not something that you eat. Instead, this is a useful tool that forces you to record everything you eat. Now be prepared for a surprise here, because if you aren't aware of what you're stuffing into your maw, you will remain in blimpdom forever. So unless you're an actor and the role requires rolls (of fat), you need to pay attention. Like the rubber band, the log forces you to become more aware of what kind of things you're vacuuming up all day long, and why you are starting to swell up like one of those inflatable ornaments that have been springing up on lawns everywhere during holidays.

And in case you get really hungry and the snapping is making you look as if you've been taken into custody one time too many, then try a light snack of ten baby carrots or cherry tomatoes. It is very important that you eat ten instead of just a few. The reason is that ten will fill you up and then you'll be able to forget about food for a while. Just one or two won't do it, and you'll still be thinking about food. I keep bowls of them around to keep me out of trouble. They are great when you desperately need to chew something, especially at the beginning of the diet.

If you use all these tricks, you'll be so busy snapping, writing, drinking, and running to the bathroom that you won't have time for snacks at all anymore!

## SURVIVAL HINTS

1. Always keep healthy snacks around that you won't get into trouble with if you eat too many. Included are hardboiled eggs, celery, cucumber slices, and, of course, the baby carrots and cherry tomatoes.

2.  Be sure to get in your quota of water when you're dieting because it really helps keep you hydrated; it also helps eliminate the fat you're burning off.

3.  Be sure to reward yourself when you reach your goal. Sometimes a picture of the reward taped to the fridge can really keep you out of trouble.

4.  Also helpful is a photo of a slim person in a bathing suit. It'll remind you that overeating and too many snacks can catch up with you!

# The No-Diet Diet

*Samantha Hearns*

I AM ON THE NO-DIET DIET, and if you are one of those people who eats only when hungry, you can be, too. You see, the No-Diet Diet covers you from every dieting street. If you happen to turn up Double Chocolate Layer Cake Lane, you will only come to find it's a dead end. Immediately turn your carcass around and hightail it out of town. When you feel the instant need to turn onto Tiramisu Terrace, your carcass alarm will wreak havoc in the lower end of your neighborhood. Now not wanting to make a spectacle out of yourself, you could just put yourself in neutral and roll off the street. But you love that neighborhood. The structures are sweet and delicate, and stopping only once to take in the sights will not be a problem, right? Wrong!

The more you tell yourself it's okay to cruise the same streets that got you into trouble in the first place, the harder you are making the no-diet diet on yourself.

On the no-diet diet you are allowed to eat anything you want. You are in control, and there are no rules to follow. There is no calorie counting, no weighing your food, no weighing yourself. The no-diet diet is a self-reliant system. You rely on yourself for your own judgment on what's right and what's wrong for you.

For me, bread and cheese have always been a weakness. There is nothing like a good crusty piece of bread topped with a slice of your favorite cheese accompanied by a glass of your favorite burgundy, nothing wrong with that, except what it does to your waistline.

On the no-diet diet, you can just say no. But if you are like most of us, "no" doesn't apply to food. On the no-diet diet, your entire source of controlling your intake, and ultimately the size of your butt, rests upon your shoulders, or maybe your legs.

So now maybe you would like to know just how this no-diet diet works? Well, listen up. It's short and sweet. *Eat only when you're hungry!* Most people eat all day long, especially when they are overweight. They eat when they're watching television, when they're talking on the phone, when they're driving their cars—they aren't paying attention to what they are consuming, and they also don't realize they're full. Why? Because their attention is elsewhere.

If you stop as soon as you are full, eating only when you are hungry has no negatives. This means you have to pay attention, and you must eat slowly enough for your head to realize that your stomach is full. Once you learn how to do this, you will never again feel the need to consume large portions because you will never be hungry. Of course, you need to eat three healthy meals a day to fuel your body, and have healthy snacks only when you really need them. And you can't do anything else while you are eating. And I mean nothing else! No watching television, no eating in the car, no talking on the phone, no reading. You must concentrate on your food, and you must take your time.

Doing this will allow you to curb your appetite forever. You'll lose pounds and turn yourself back into the shapely hottie you once were and want to be once again. And then you'll be able to take a stroll on Romance Road, and have a ride on Hot Honey Hill—all because you went on the no-diet diet!

**5**

# When You're
# Dieting and Dating

## Dieting with Mr. Wrong
Carole A. Daley

## My Date with a Dieter
Walter C. Hahn

## Looking for Mr. Goodybar
Barbara Dawson

# Sanity Quiz

You met your mate at a support group for dieters. On your diets and otherwise, the two of you were having a great relationship—but then he suddenly started shoveling it in like never before.

Do you

A. tell him you're sorry, but the size of your butt is more important to you than he is
B. help him make it over his hurdle
C. find a non-gorging mate and dump Mr. Eats-Too-Much
D. stick to your diet plan and hope he finds his way back to his

If you're dieting and dating and you answered yes to any of these questions, then you really need to check out the following stories. For those of us who have been diet-derailed by a date, there's solace ahead.

# Dieting with Mr. Wrong

*Carole A. Daley*

A HALF-GALLON OF ice cream never made it through the night at my parents' house. When I was growing up, it was unthinkable not to have dessert every night. A meal was what stood between dessert and me. At my Los Angeles high school, lunch was two cartons of whole milk and two candy bars. California, always a leader, stocked its schools with candy machines long before the rest of the country started fattening up the student population. I went from a skinny kid to an overweight teenager in a few weeks.

My college years were my yo-yo dieting years. I lost and regained the same ten pounds a dozen times. After graduation, I joined a management-training program and found myself in a chic Beverly Hills office. With few exceptions, everyone was impossibly thin. Their tiny cinched waists contrasted with my ever-expanding waistline. In spite of my five-foot three-inch frame, I had entered the world of double-digit sizes. The only other heavy woman was pregnant, and she was my lunch partner.

Besides our love of large lunches, the other thing my pregnant desk mate and I had in common was our disdain for Matt, who, we assumed, was the office "boy toy." At office parties, all the other women flocked to Matt like hungry baby birds vying for mama bird's attention. Matt was charming, handsome, and he exuded a rich frat boy's confidence. Not my type.

I thought my type was Nick. One afternoon as I was trying to stay awake in front of a pile of mind-numbing reports, a trim, well-dressed man looked into the office. Quickly nudging my quietly snoozing pregnant pal, I asked her who the Adonis was.

"Oh, that's Nick Q. He's a marketing bigwig, works on the top floor. Uh, thanks for waking me up," she sighed as she straightened up in her chair. "He looks pretty intense," she added.

"And unattainable," I mumbled.

Never one to let ceremony or simple introductions stand in my way, I called Nick. On the pretext of trainee enthusiasm, I asked him to lunch. Nick accepted.

That night, I bought a silk suit that I couldn't afford on my trainee salary. I also began my standard "lose weight fast" dinner, a six-pack of diet Dr. Pepper. On the appointed day, Matt appeared at my desk and cheerfully announced, "Nick can't make it, but I'd love to take you to lunch."

As it turned out, Matt worked for Nick. Not knowing how to decline his eager invitation, I sat through lunch with barely concealed disappointment. After lunch, I called Nick and asked for a new date. "Well, I do need a lap counter this weekend," he offered.

"A lap counter?" I thought to myself. I couldn't imagine what he meant, but I told him I would be happy to be his lap counter.

A lap counter turned out to be just that—someone counting each lap of the track as the runner completed it. Nick was training to run in a charity event. I suited up in the only thing I had that looked remotely athletic—a dark blue nylon warm-up suit, never worn, that my mother had given me for my birthday. Nick equipped me with a stopwatch, but I quickly lost track of his time and laps. Nick was not amused.

Running six days a week wasn't his only exercise. He also swam laps on the weekends. Eventually, Nick couldn't pass up my adulation and we became a couple. But everything was on his terms. I joined him in his running and swimming obsessions. At first, I wasn't good at either activity. I had never run more than the mandatory mile for the President's Physical Fitness Test in elementary school (which I minimally passed), and my swimming was rudimentary. No one had ever accused me of being an athlete. I entered a ten-kilometer race Nick had casually mentioned. It was my first race and I finished dead last.

But persistence paid off and the side effect of all that exercise was shrinking thighs. The other benefit was the fuel. Nick knew the restaurants that served huge plates of steamed vegetables on brown rice covered with a blanket of grated cheese. We ate salads with dressing on the side. Fast food never passed Nick's lips, but he shared my persistent sweet tooth.

One day as I was looking for a rubber band in Nick's "junk drawer" I picked up a snapshot of a round-faced, beyond-plump man. "Who's the chubby chap?" I asked.

Plucking it from my fingers, Nick barked, "Me!"

Months later, I discovered his other secret. One night, he didn't show up for our date. The next morning, I ran down to the ocean and clocked in extra miles to mask my distress. The story he told when he called was easier to endure because I was still feeling the after effects of a great run. I also found out that "I need some time to myself" really means "I've met someone else." Indeed, Nick had met someone at the swim club.

The relationship went from bad to worse. The break-up was brutal and prolonged, but I kept running. And I came out the winner: I was twenty-five pounds lighter, and I had adopted a new set of diet rules that have persisted to this day.

## SURVIVAL HINTS

1. *The Nonfat Rule.* I choose the nonfat alternatives whenever possible. Nonfat milk and yogurt are staples in my refrigerator.

2. *The Water Rule.* I buy 1.5-liter bottles of water by the case and drink one bottle every day. Yes, I visit the bathroom every few minutes, but I stop drinking water by 8:30 p.m. so that I'll make it to the morning without a potty break. When I'm cold, I drink hot water.

3. *The Twenty-Minute Rule.* When the tug of the chocolate cake becomes too strong, I set the timer for twenty minutes and remove myself from the cake's sphere of influence. And, just as the diet gurus promise, my brain catches up with my stomach and the craving disappears.

4. *The Wise Consumer Rule.* I read food labels as if they contained the secret of life. Knowing there are more grams of sugar in a "nutrition" bar than a scoop of ice cream does make a difference in my choices.

5. *The Dessert Rule.*   I try not to substitute dessert for a meal. I love myself enough to reach for the salad.

6. *The Portion Rule.*   It doesn't take a math whiz to figure out that the portions served in most eating establishments are enough for two meals. Doggie bags are my friends.

7. *The Dressing Rule.*   I always order salad dressing on the side.

8. *The Exercise Rule.*   I eat much better on the days that I exercise. I don't know why, and I don't care why. I make it my goal to exercise every day.

9. *The "Identify the Craving" Rule.*   Social anxiety? Trying to meet a deadline? Need comfort? Okay, I've got an oral fixation—I admit it. But it seems that everyone in America has an oral fixation, so I've got lots of company. I reach for my water bottle and a box of crackers (no hydrogenated oils, of course). In my pre-Nick days, when I felt ill at ease at a party or anywhere else, I'd dig into the brownie bites. It works just as well to stuff carrot and celery sticks in my mouth, and I feel a lot better during and after the minicrisis.

10. *The "I'm In Charge" Rule.*   I'm in charge of what I eat, unless the ice cream starts calling my name from the freezer, then I remember Rule Number 3.

I can't always control my calorie intake, but I can control my calorie burning. My motto is this: "No steps too steep, no parking spot too far." Why drive if I can walk? When I'm bored or tired, I go jogging. I've expanded my repertoire beyond Nick's simple regime. There are more forms of vigorous exercise than I'll ever be able to try in one lifetime. I've fallen in and out of love with cycling classes, interval training, power pump, Pilates, and yoga, and when I broke my foot, I signed up for water aerobics.

Exercise is a gift I can share with friends or enjoy alone. As for my love life after Nick, Matt showed up on my doorstep and it turned out that he was more than just a pretty face. He, too, is an avid jogger, but he doesn't like to swim—just as well!

# My Date with a Dieter

*Walter C. Hahn*

SHE WAS BEAUTIFUL in that slim, sleek style that some women have. Tall, light-brown hair, beautiful face, long neck, high cheekbones. Wide-set blue eyes, perfect nose. She was shy, but articulate and nearly brilliant when she spoke. I liked the way her face lit up when she smiled. A true beauty. Even better, she seemed largely unaware of her beauty.

It was a first date. We dined in a very expensive high-end place—the restaurant had a rooftop view of Chicago, and the lake was gorgeous that evening. We each had a glass of pinot grigio, and then the menus came.

I glanced down the list and picked out a big fat steak with all the trimmings. Then I noticed the raised eyebrows of my companion. "See anything you like?" I asked.

"Well," she replied, "I like fish and the Arctic char looks interesting, as does the bronzino, but they both have sauce on them, and I never eat sauce." I grimaced inwardly and thought, "Oh, joy. She's one of those sauce-on-the-side types who eats naked salad— 'Dressing on the side, please!'" God, help me!

The waiter noticed her expression of distress and asked whether he could answer any questions. She told him of her sauce aversion, and the waiter reassured her that whatever she chose could be prepared any way she wished. "Would you like the fish grilled?" he asked. "There is normally just a tiny bit of marinade on the fish to keep it moist during the grilling." "Oh," she replied. "Can it be prepared without the marinade?" "Of course, if that's your preference, Ma'am," he said earnestly, but with a twitch of concern. "Yes, then I'd like the char, please," she asserted.

She went on and ordered the salad, dressing on the side, just as I had predicted, and a glass of water with lemon. I ordered my decadent steak dinner, and noticed her slight tremor as I requested both sour cream and butter for the potato, as well as chunky blue cheese dressing for my salad, not to mention the escargots en croute as an appetizer, which, of course, she virtuously declined.

When the appetizer came, I offered to share it; she shook her head and warded it off with a raised palm— just the way a school crossing guard stops traffic. Next came the salads. She zealously squirted lemon juice on hers, and a dash of vinegar—that was all. At least it wasn't dry. Then she picked off the gorgeous sliver of reggiano parmigiana cheese that came atop the greens and cast it aside. My heart broke a little.

Finally, our main course arrived. My platter was luscious—it looked as if it had come right out of a photo shoot for *Gourmet* magazine. Hers, on the other hand, looked anemic. It was sad. Plain. Boring. Probably devoid of flavor. At least there was a wedge of lemon on the side, and some spinach.

I dug in and devoured a corner of my filet mignon, and asked her if she liked her dinner. "Lovely," she replied, as she tasted the plank set before her. What a waste of culinary opportunity, I thought. But to each his or her own, and she certainly was thin.

We talked about the view, the lake, the weather, the service in the restaurant. I raved about my steak. She smiled politely. I asked her what her favorite food was, thinking that if there was a second date, I'd try to find something more to her liking. "Oh, I'll eat anything," she replied.

As we worked our way through the main course, I noticed that she had cut her fish in half and had moved it, along with half the buttered spinach, to the other side of her plate. Curious, I asked her whether something was wrong with the other half. She replied, "I'm on a diet. I gained a pound and a half last month, and I must deal with it immediately. So I halve all my portions, especially in restaurants, and skip desserts."

"Oh," I replied. My timing obviously wasn't so great with this dinner date, and I thought ruefully of the double chocolate cheesecake that was the restaurant's specialty dessert.

"How often do you diet?" I asked politely. "Almost all the time," she responded. "It's a way of life, otherwise I'll turn out to be fat. Three pounds can become thirteen before you know it."

"But you don't have a weight problem!" I protested. "Ah, but one can't be too careful," she said firmly. "I've invested years in keeping in shape, so I don't want to mess it up now—because it'll only get harder, and studies show that if you have to go on more than one or two major diets during your adult life, you can have serious health repercussions, and I don't want that to happen."

"Well," I replied, "I guess you know what you're doing." I thought of my rotund German mother and aunts, their platters of wursts, their bowls of mashed potatoes and sauerkraut, their sauce-infused delicacies, their strudels; I realized then that a future with this lovely lady would be impossible unless we brought Lean Cuisine along to feed her.

The waiter stopped by to see how everything was. "Great," I replied. He then spied her divided meal: "Miss, is anything wrong with your dinner? I could take it back and get you something else if you aren't happy with the fish," he said with concern. "Oh, no, it's very good. I'm just not that hungry. Would you wrap it, please?" I was still eating my steak, but what could I do? "Would you wrap mine, too? It's really a big portion. Thanks a lot," I said with some frustration. As we sat uncomfortably trying to think of something to talk about, the waiter reappeared.

"Can I interest you in dessert today?" he asked, tremulously. "Oh, none for me, thanks. Just more water," said the queen of dieters, Miss Sans Saucey.

Well, I thought. This isn't going so well anyway, so what the heck. And I was still hungry! "I'll have the double chocolate cheesecake, please, and an Irish coffee, thanks." "Very good choice, sir," grinned the waiter as he zipped efficiently away. My date's eyes nearly popped. "You're going to have both?" she said, disapprovingly. I simply nodded slowly.

Dessert arrived, I enjoyed it. It was a huge wedge of dark chocolate cheesecake, chocolate chunks laced throughout, and topped by a fluffy mound of freshly whipped cream. Now I decided to be vengeful.

I described the texture of the cheesecake, the consistency of the whipped cream, the richness of the chocolate, and soon the diet queen looked as if she was going to faint from her efforts to restrain herself. Finally, I offered her a bite. "Oh, good heavens no!" she cried. "I couldn't possibly!" "You sure?" I asked, temptingly. I held out a morsel on the sterling silver fork. "Can't you smell that incredible chocolate flavor?" I asked. I kept the fork extended to her, a big smile on my face. "It's really, really amazing," I tempted.

At last, she relented. Her eyes were beginning to water, and I'm sure she would have begun drooling next. "Okay, maybe just a little." Before I knew it, she'd eaten three-quarters of the cheesecake and was chattering happily about her job, her family, and her hopes and dreams. We were married within the year.

I guess the moral of the story is that it's great to be careful about what you eat, but sometimes you just have to enjoy what lands in your lap!

## SURVIVAL HINTS

1. It really does work to cut your portions in half, especially when you're first starting to eat out while you're dieting.
2. Drinking water helps to keep you from overeating.
3. Lemon or vinegar is a great tasting substitute for salad dressing, which is high in both fat and calories. Low fat cottage cheese also works really well.
4. When you're eating out, substitute a fresh vegetable for the potato, rice or pasta.
5. Once in a while, you can have a taste of something forbidden—it can keep you from bingeing later.

# Looking for Mr. Goodybar

*Barbara Dawson*

I WAS ON A HUNT for the man of my dreams when I encountered Mr. Goodybar. He was everything I had ever wanted. Smart, sexy, of sound mind, and so much like me that it was scary. He loved everything I loved, right down to the double-butter popcorn at the theatre. We ate, we drank, and we sang and danced together. We indulged to excess. I was so happy. After twelve years of looking for Mr. Right, I had finally found him—or so I thought.

You see, with this love came a price: my body. I had turned myself from being slightly overweight (I had toted around an extra ten pounds) to way overweight

(I discovered I was dragging around my butt, which was now at knee-level). But it was hard for me to realize where the problem had originated.

Before Mr. Goodybar arrived, I was depressed, and I blamed that depression on my lack of companionship. I thought that if I had a man in my life, I would not be sitting alone stuffing my face but instead would be out and about, being wined and dined.

And for the first few months that was how it went. We ate out every night and followed dinner with a movie or dancing. Then we went home and enjoyed each other until the wee hours of the morning. But as time went on we began to get lazy. We started ordering dinner in or, worse yet, cooking it ourselves and throwing portion control right out the window. The dancing had turned into television and our other delightful extra curricular exercise had turned into a slice of cake or a king-sized candy bar.

This wasn't what I had bargained for, but I was in love. How do you separate your love for food from your love for your man and his companionship? Now I had quite the struggle in front of me, and I didn't know how to approach the subject. For Mr. Goodybar was my first true love.

I had always kept track of my weight, ever since I was a teenager. I had gone from fat to thin many times, and I always was able to see the root of the problem. But this time was different. This wasn't about just me; it was also about the man I was in love with, who, by the way, had gained as much as I had, plus one. We were falling apart at the hand of food. Everything we had enjoyed together had been shot to hell. We didn't dine out, we didn't dance, we didn't go to the theatre; and the last thing either of us wanted to do with these fat bodies was to get naked.

I had to broach the delicate subject, and with caution. "I think we have a problem," I said. Then he looked into my eyes, as sweetly and sensually as he had on many other nights, and said, "What, are we out of ice cream? I'll go this time." Since becoming Mr. and Ms. Fat Stuff, we had taken turns running out for the food. "No," I said. "That's not it. We are overeating and losing what once was a good life for us. Look at me. Did I look like this when you met me?" I stood up and swept my hands from head to toe.

He didn't know what to say, so I replied for him: "No, I didn't. And you didn't either!" He looked down to his own belly and said, "I guess we got a bit out of hand."

"Just a bit misguided," I said. Mr. Goodybar and I went on a diet that day, and it wasn't easy because we had fallen into a pattern. But people can change patterns, and that is exactly what we did. We adjusted and readjusted until we fell into what worked for us as a couple. Soon, instead of overindulging in food, we were back to overindulging in each other.

## SURVIVAL HINTS

1. Sometimes dieting is better if you do it with a partner, and you'll have something to focus on together as you plan the meals, shop for the ingredients, and prepare the food.

2. Don't be afraid to tell your significant other what's on your mind, especially if it involves changing the way you approach food together. Many new couples gain weight because so much of their social lives involve food. It's helpful to address food and diet issues before they snowball.

**6**

# When You're Dieting with a Partner

# Sanity Quiz

It's Saturday night and you're dining with your other half at your favorite little bistro. The waiter is waiting to take your order. All day you have been craving lasagna. As you begin to order your heart's desire, your other heart's desire cuts you off in mid-sentence and suggests that you eat something less fattening.

Do you

A. tell him to shut up and worry about his own order
B. speak louder than your other half and order your lasagna anyway
C. cave in and eat a light meal
D. eat the light meal and an even larger-than-lasagna dessert

If you answered yes to any of these questions, you need to read on!

# Spring Cleaning

*M. M. Patterson*

I KNEW FROM ITS NAME that a diet called "The Cleanse" wouldn't be easy, but I agreed to give it a try to support my husband, who had heard great things about it from coworkers. Extra and consistent energy levels were promised, as was the vaguely attractive though somewhat frightening notion of "clarity of thought." We were game to try anything once, but let's call a spade a spade: This was colon cleansing. This wouldn't be pretty. Still, a bodily spring clean sounded doable, if not exactly fun. And we wouldn't miss the pounds that we might shed as a happy byproduct of our clean-eating efforts.

"The Cleanse" would last three weeks. During Week 1, our menu would be simple, the simplest it had ever been: fruits and vegetables, warm water, peppermint tea, and strange-sounding all-natural supplements that would help us digest and expel what little variety *would* go in our mouths. Digest and expel: Words to live by. No one said we'd need to stay near a bathroom at all times, but we imagined the worst and didn't plan any long-distance travel.

During Week 2, we would be allowed to add grains to the mix: brown rice, nuts, and seeds. A herbivore's dream.

Week 3 would bring the by-then much-needed addition of some protein—beans or fish. Oh, joy!

The more I found out about the details of this undertaking, the more I questioned the wisdom of my giving it a whirl. Doctor's orders were one thing, but I didn't recall that "for better or for worse" includes suffering just for kicks.

As our "diet start date" approached, my anxiety and sarcasm grew. I found myself obsessing about what we *would* be allowed to eat and, in the sarcasm department, about how regular we would surely become. Though my husband distracted himself by shopping and preparing, I found myself savoring "the last cup of coffee," "the last cookie," "the last bite of chicken." For a week before we began, each meal was like the last one in death row.

But time marches on when it's not actually your last day on death row. Our start date arrived, bright and sunny, despite the dark clouds gathering in our kitchen.

⟜⟞

Everyone has a breaking point, and Day 4 was mine. I never thought I'd miss salt so very much. I desperately needed more than the leek-and-carrot gruel my husband prepared for dinner. A chunk of crusty bread would have been a good start. I desperately wanted a few of the buttered tortellini our kids were happily feasting on. Even one—just to test that they were al dente—would have been a real treat. And I desperately needed a break from the constant talk of cleansing foods. Let's be honest: Colon cleansing isn't sexy. No loving couple can talk about it and expect to be turned on. But what else was there?

And so it was for the remainder of that difficult first week. Day 8 arrived and we added nuts and seeds, but let's face it, nuts and seeds are bird food. They might do the trick of filling you up in great quantity but they are not—by any stretch of the imagination—satisfying. Brown rice was a welcome starch, but I would never describe it as delicious or complex. It's rice, but brown. Without butter and without salt, it tastes like, well, rice.

It was about this time—Day 8 or 9 if memory serves—that the distinct difference in metabolism between my husband and me started to become apparent. You see, whereas I seemed to be barely hanging on, my husband had hit his stride. He was eating what I was eating and expelling as often as I was expelling (often!) and he was starting to feel fantastic, energetic, spry. He was always unflappable and even-keeled, but he seemed just a little more bright-eyed and perky every day. Strangely so. And he'd lost weight—perhaps five pounds. "Good for you," I said rather glumly as he jumped enthusiastically from the scale. I really wanted to be happy for him but couldn't quite summon the energy to be anything but a little bitter.

And who could blame me? I hadn't lost an ounce and was feeling sluggish and a little bit empty all the time. I was becoming more and more unhappy about my pledge of support on this crazy diet, and I was also finding it increasingly hard to grin and bear it. I wasn't ravenous. I wasn't craving anything specific. I just needed more food, more *real* food.

Most of all, I needed my food-loving gourmand of a husband back on my side. The man standing in his place was irrationally happy and gung-ho. Every comment about how great he was feeling, how much energy he had, and how sharp his focus was made me angrier and angrier. I imagined I knew what it must be like when a loved one joined a cult. He seemed lost to me forever. And I told him so. We didn't speak for the better part of Day 10.

But a day and a half later, I started to feel better . . . so much better that I, too, had more spring in my step and more energy throughout the day. For lack of a better way to put it, I simply felt light. And no surprise—after all, I wasn't eating much of substance—I *was* lighter. When I checked on Day 13, I had lost six pounds! Still ahead of me in the weight loss department, though neck and neck in the cheeriness race, my husband had lost nine pounds. Cleansed? Sure, you could say that, too. I was eating nuts and seeds and fruit by the fistful; I do believe I tried every exotic vegetable in the market. I certainly had never been so productive in the bathroom!

But strange things started to happen: I found myself uncharacteristically patient with my children. I had a new-found and unusually high tolerance for whining and back talk. I was oh-so-Zen about life.

And then the real weirdness: I found myself considering bikinis in catalogs for the first time in fifteen years. I ordered one right away in my old size, too. Red, thank you very much.

What's the old saying? No good deed goes unpunished? Or perhaps more fitting for the purposes of this little narrative: All good things must come to an end.

Indeed, by the middle of the third cleansing week, and despite the addition of some welcome protein to our diet, our respective highs came crashing down to new lows. How quickly we had come back down to Earth, and at the same time, too! We'd lost some serious weight (seventeen pounds total) but we were exhausted by the effort and cranky with a constant low-grade hunger. And our genuine good cheer had gone sour like the milk left untouched for weeks in the fridge.

So, as any red-blooded, hungry, and embittered team would do, we began to plot our revenge.

In place of talking about how we would stew, roast, boil, steam, or bake the next batch of vegetables, instead of discussing the merits of currants over raisins when poached with pears in water, instead of comparing the nature and frequency of our trips to the can, we started to talk about what we would eat when we could eat what we wanted! We imagined the filet mignon we would put on the grill, and the butter shallot sauce we'd spoon over it. We dreamed up thick and creamy pasta sauces. We considered buying a bread maker so that we'd be able to enjoy the aroma of baking bread all day. We bought a case of wine and selected the bottle we'd open at the end of the week.

We cut out the most decadent recipes from cooking magazines and readied ourselves to cook lavishly.

And then the day arrived. We could put our plans into action. And we did. And we did some more. You'd have thought we'd learned our lesson about going to extremes, but we were making up for lost time here, don't forget. I am not ashamed to say it now: I had never and have not since eaten such a variety of colon-clogging foods in so short a time and with such gusto. That day was heaven.

The next day, of course, was hell. Uncomfortable, sluggish, cranky-for-a-whole-new-gassy-reason kind of hell.

Of course, the moral of the story is that going to extremes with food is punishable by extreme discomfort at either end of the belly spectrum. Up-down, up-down, clean-clog, clean-clog: The digestive system can take only so much stress! Moderation is the best medicine, and spring cleaning, it turns out, is a concept best left to closets! Which is right where that red bikini is stored now. Better luck next year.

# Dieting with Grace

*Evelyn M. Fazio*

WHEN I WAS ABOUT SIXTEEN, I decided to lose weight. I had been a skinny little kid, so skinny that the relatives used to comment, and I never wanted to eat. And I was always sick—lots of sore throats, tonsillitis, colds, and so on, which probably contributed to my lack of appetite. My parents actually used to bribe me to eat—make bets, cook my favorite foods, offer snacks at bedtime. They tried everything.

After my tonsillectomy, the stream of weight-inducing goodies didn't end with the surgery. Then puberty hit and I began to take on ballast. By the time I was fourteen, I ended up weighing about twenty pounds more than I should have. Now sixteen, I needed to do something about it, and fast.

That fateful summer, Grace, our neighbor across the street, a big lady, and a retired nurse, went on a diet. She stopped by one afternoon with her jumbo German shepherd and announced that she'd gone on a new diet. It was the first one that made you drink a ton of water, and it was called the Stillman Diet. It was designed by a doctor, and they gave you sample menus, and all kinds of good suggestions for taking off the extra poundage. She'd already lost three pounds!

I told her I wanted to try it too, so she photocopied all the information from some magazine article. "We can be diet buddies," she said. I was on my way.

Having been so skinny for so long, I had become used to eating whatever I wanted. But now, for the first time ever, I turned a blind eye to the amazing array of delicious foods flowing from my parents' kitchen. I welded myself to the exact protocols of the diet. I ate a half an orange and a slice of toast for breakfast; lunch was vegetarian vegetable soup and an apple; dinner a hamburger patty with mustard and a cup of consommé. Dessert no longer existed, and I didn't miss it.

You had to drink eight big glasses of water a day to keep you feeling full and to help keep you hydrated and eliminate lost fat, and you couldn't stray far from a bathroom at first!

That summer, the diet worked its magic and I stuck to it like a barnacle on a ship. Nothing, and I *mean* nothing, deterred me from my goal. Soon my clothes were getting loose. Soon I needed a whole new wardrobe! Soon I could wear pants and not look like something that should have Goodyear printed on it.

Next, Grace informed me that I needed to exercise or I'd be flabby. Ugh. What a thought. I didn't like sports and had always been inactive, preferring to read and draw than run around playing baseball or join in the other activities the neighborhood kids got into. I was the artistic, literary type, and it wasn't good for my metabolism.

So I started walking everywhere: to the mall, to the magazine store, to the supermarket—wherever I had to go. Next thing you know, I was walking four miles to the orthodontist, three miles to see a movie, and so on. It was great—and if my feet gave out, I'd call home for a ride. My legs looked good, and I was getting thinner and thinner. Soon I was ready to go back to school, and Grace was more excited for me than I was.

First day back in class, nobody recognized me.

But it wasn't just the weight. Because I was spending less time eating and more on my appearance, I had learned to wrestle my thick curly black hair into submission. I went from bride of Frankenstein to the style that we all wanted—smooth and straight. I was fine as long as it didn't rain! Next, my parents insisted that I wear contact lenses, then the orthodontist surprised me by removing my braces ahead of schedule. A pair of tweezers took care of my aggressively overgrown eyebrows, and style magazines taught me what I needed to know about makeup. It was my own brand of makeover, and I looked different—and unrecognizable—even to my friends.

And I stuck to my diet even then. Meanwhile, Grace was like a one-woman cheering squad, coming over to check on my progress and congratulating me on my efforts. She was losing, too, and also needed new clothes. She even treated herself to a new haircut.

Grace ended up losing thirty pounds. Even her dog, Mickey, looked thinner. And we were both really glad to have had each other for dieting partners because it clearly helped us both stick to our plans. Even today when I decide to lose a few pounds, I think of Grace and say thank you!

## SURVIVAL HINTS

1. Exercise is critical. Start out slowly, even if you only walk around the block once a day to begin with; work your way up to thirty minutes, then forty-five. Soon you'll be sleek as a cat, and everyone else will be hissing with jealousy!

2. Water helps keep off weight because it helps cut the cravings, fills you up, and keeps you hydrated, making you feel well and energetic. It's also good for your skin, making it look younger and smoother. This, too, will make everyone around you take notice. And then they'll all be carrying around bottles of water after they've finished hissing again!

3. Portion control is important—don't overdo anything, no matter how much the devil on your shoulder whispers in your ear: "Aw, go ahead . . . it's just a little taste." Give him a swat and send him reeling, and then stick to your plan.

4. Give your stomach a chance to catch up with your mouth; wait at least fifteen to twenty minutes for another helping of anything but carrots and celery because sometimes it takes a while to feel full, even though you've had plenty to eat.

5. Keep bags of healthy snacks around—small carrots, cherry tomatoes, celery, dry roasted almonds (unsalted only!). Better to eat some of these than drink a pint of Ben & Jerry's, and you won't need a shoehorn to put on your pants!

6. Stay away from sugar and all those fake sweeteners. After a day or two, you won't miss them, and you will start to realize how good things taste without the extra "help."

# Jack the Dieter

*William Tucker*

MY PARTNER JACK is a diet lunatic. He is the most health-conscious person I know, always worried about exercise and his intake and output, not to mention my intake and output. You see, Jack is a real character. Not only is he concerned about his own weight and appearance but now he has taken me on as a challenge, and a mighty one at that. He watches everything I eat as if he were my mother and I his child. Now, I don't mind this much because there is little chance I'll do it by myself. I have never been one to count calories or weigh my food, and that just may be how I ended up with these extra thirty pounds to begin with.

Jack and I always dine together, mostly at outdoor cafés and bistros, where we can sit comfortably and go over the day's events while picking the menus apart as much as possible. Jack is notorious for this.

"I think I'll have the pasta," I said. Jack cleared his throat, rolled his eyes and lifted his menu to cover the disapproval on his face. "What?" I said. "Nothing, nothing," he replied, raising his hands as if to ward off an argument. "What's wrong with the pasta?" I asked. "You just had pasta the night before last. Don't you think something a bit lighter, better for you, would be more appropriate?" he responded. "What would you suggest?" I asked.

"The spinach salad looks delightful, accompanied by a glass of spring water with a fresh slice of lemon. The perfect meal. You know you are supposed to be watching your weight, dear," he said. Jack and I have been together for years, and I know his concern for me comes out of love. But my God, can he be a nag.

To further avoid escalation into a more dangerous argument, I conceded. We both ordered the spinach salad and spring water, and Jack smiled beatifically the whole time I ate because he had won, once again. Well, dinner came and went, and then Jack said, "Let's finish up by splitting a piece of pumpkin torte."

Dessert has always been Jack's downfall. No matter how much he watches everything we both eat, his sweet tooth has always had a way of sneaking up on him. "Pumpkin torte?" I asked. "You didn't want me to have pasta, but you are going to get pumpkin torte? You don't really want that torte, do you?" "I guess not," he said sheepishly.

As usual, Jack and I had once again saved each other from countless extra calories using our usual approach of mutual nagging and pestering—but one that worked for us. Jack saved me from the pasta and I saved him from the pumpkin torte. And just to get even for depriving me of that bowl of pasta, I never told him about the big piece of spinach that had lodged itself on his "too sweet to tell him" tooth.

## SURVIVAL HINTS

1. A dieting partner is often a plus as long as you both are on the same diet; you can then monitor and help each other choose carefully what you stuff into your mouths.

2. Be sure that the competition stays friendly or else you could sabotage yourself and your diet partner. Try not to resort to overly aggressive behavior, which can backfire, and nobody else wants to see your fur flying, especially in a restaurant!

# My Challenge Diet

*Judy Banta*

WHEN I WAS THIRTY-TWO years old, I gained eighty pounds. Why? Because I had a baby. He weighed ten pounds, but at least sixty of the eighty were now mine. I looked like a small planet. Forty-inch thighs, and don't even ask about the waist and hips. It was bad, very bad. Not to mention the ripples and dimples.

Because of my rotund state, I could hardly bend over and pick up a piece of lint, much less anything else. I couldn't see my feet, or my knees, or anything below the bulge. They may as well have been in another ZIP code.

Finally, after coming around a corner, I saw myself unexpectedly in a full-length mirror in my friend's high-rise apartment lobby. I wondered who that blimp was, then nearly shrieked from horror when I realized that it was time to take action. Or a diet pill. Or something. But the Orca imitation had to stop, and now.

The first thing I did was throw away all the cake, cookies, candy, and other goodies people kept bringing me when our baby was born. Second, I announced that I was starting a diet, and I challenged anyone who was brave enough to a contest—whoever lost fifty pounds first would be taken out to dinner in the best restaurant in town—paid for by the loser!

My brother-in-law, Ralph, Orca-esque himself, couldn't pass it up. He was gigunda. Made me look almost svelte (I said almost!). He had a sixty-inch waist, a twenty-five-inch neck, and he hadn't seen his feet in about twenty years.

So now I was motivated. Orca-Ralph had always loved to annoy me, and he went out of his way to be a pest, in a teasingly irritating way. He wasn't a bad person, just a pain. Anyway, now Ralph was going to lose fifty pounds before I could? Not a chance in hell.

The first thing I did after Ralph accepted my challenge was to start writing down everything I put in my mouth. It was the only way to understand what was going on, and how all this fat "happened." I was shocked and horrified after only a few hours. I was the McCormick Reaper of eaters. Anything that got into my path was mowed down in seconds. Nothing was safe, even food I didn't like.

Next I concentrated on what was making me eat. Was it that I was tired? Was it because the baby kept me up half the night and I wanted to feel better? Was it because I felt as if there was no hope of ever becoming thin?

I began to realize that food was a substitute for rest, a sedative for frustration, and a pacifier that sometimes lasted only a few seconds. Whatever it was, armed with my new knowledge and insights, I took the bull by the horns.

Now I vowed to eat tiny portions, to drink water, to eat only at mealtimes—no in between snacks—and to go for walks with the baby in the stroller—all to use up some calories and get a little exercise. The tiny portions ended up being small instead of tiny, but they helped. I also stayed away from pasta, bread, potatoes, and all the starchy stuff I'd been living on. Next, I gave up dessert entirely—and if I wanted something for a treat, I'd have a cup of hot chocolate or a piece of fruit and a cup of green tea.

After about two weeks, I noticed that my elephant-sized pants were getting loose! I was so surprised. I hadn't really been focusing on what was going on because I was too busy writing things down, not to mention taking care of a baby.

Little by little, I shrank down almost to a normal size. Meanwhile, I hadn't seen Ralph in about a month. He showed up at my house one day with a big chocolate cake. "Neither one of us is ever going to get thin," he said, clearly oblivious to my now much smaller size, "so we might as well enjoy it—we can't help being what we are." I wanted borrow a forklift from Costco and throw him out the door!

Instead, I made a pot of coffee, sat down at the table, and said, "Ralph, if you want to look like a beached whale for the rest of your life, go right ahead. But I intend to be thin again, whether you like it or not. So have a piece of cake, and take the rest of it with you or it's going into the garbage." Ralph dropped his fork in surprise and stopped eating.

"You're right," he said. "I almost sabotaged both of us." I took the cake and wrapped it up, then stuck it in the freezer. "We can thaw it out when we both reach our goal," I told him. We drank our coffee and a chastened Ralph went home.

About six months passed. I could finally fit into my pre-baby clothes. The walking had helped shed the blubber, and I started to look like the slim woman I had once been. Ralph, meanwhile, had lost quite a bit, too, and his doctor was stunned when his blood pressure dropped as well. He still had a long way to go, but he was at least getting there.

Finally, the big weigh-in took place. Everyone gathered around the scale in the kitchen. First Ralph, then me. To our stunned surprise, we had both lost exactly fifty pounds!

Laughing until our cheeks hurt, we vowed to have that dinner the following weekend, but minus the bread, the pasta, and the dessert—but we would have that slice of chocolate cake when we got home!

## SURVIVAL HINTS

1. Keep a food diary to help show where you're going astray. You'll be surprised at what you've been packing away with hardly a thought.
2. Try to focus on what's motivating you to eat at times other than at mealtimes. You might eat when you are frustrated, angry, or depressed; if so, there are better ways to cope with these feelings, which will only grow worse if you are overweight.
3. Don't let anyone sabotage you, no matter who they are. Try to sort out what may be motivating the person who offers another helping to a dieter, and don't let it or your saboteur get in your way

or derail you. The offer may be well-intentioned, but it can ruin your diet.

4. Try dieting with a partner, or challenge someone to lose the same amount of weight in a specific amount of time. This can keep your hand out of the snack bowl and your fingerprints off the fridge door handle, especially if you keep a photo of the challenger right on the door so that you don't "forget"!

5. Don't forget to enjoy your reward, even if it's chocolate cake! You can always cut a smaller piece than you used to eat. Just don't send yourself into a sugar-induced orbit from the shock!

**7**

# When You're Diet Challenged

# Sanity Quiz

You've been warned about your blood sugar. The doctor is watching you closely. You feel like a microbe under a slide. Just when you've been making progress and are seriously trying to stick to your diet, you are notified that your boss will be feted for his twenty-fifth anniversary on the job with a lavish buffet at the most exclusive restaurant in town, the one that's notorious for its decadent desserts. It's a command performance.

Do you

A. congratulate him—but pass on the offer
B. go, but bypass the buffet table
C. eat before you go
D. go stuff your face and say to hell with the doctor

If you answered yes to any of these questions, then you need some extra help and advice. Read on and see how these folks managed.

# I Was a Sleep Eater

*E. J. Bowe*

I WAS FAT. There was no doubt about it. *Fat.* Somewhere in my life I had lost control and had gained a lot of weight. All of which took up residence in my hind quarters and thighs. My doctor had put me on several diets, all to no avail. I went from a size 6 to a size 14 in two years. I couldn't see what I was doing wrong. I was exercising, eating less, and watching everything I did. But still, I was gaining weight and a lot of it.

I was not sure about what to do. I even considered surgery. It was a last resort, and one that I do not agree with (I've heard the horror stories), but I was at a dead end and desperate. If I wanted to lose weight, I had to do something.

My friend Sandy, at a local overeaters' support group, asked me whether I had ever hired a weight guard. Unfamiliar with the term, I said no, and she went on to explain. Weight guards are coaches who move in with you for a week at a time and watch everything you do. They assess your problem and try to put you back on track. This was a welcome opportunity; anything to avoid surgery.

Sandy gave me the name and contact information for Weight-Guards and away I went. The next day, a woman called Miriam moved in with me. She was tall and skinny and everything I used to be and wanted to be again. Day one came and went, and Miriam found nothing to squawk about. She said that as far as she could see, I was following my diet perfectly. That is, until about midnight.

While Miriam was asleep on the couch, I came through the living room on my way to the kitchen— my ultimate gorging ground. Dropping the peanut butter jar in my eating frenzy, I woke her up. There I was in the kitchen, with most if not all of the fattening foods in the house placed on the table, shoveling them in as if I had never eaten before. Then Miriam yelled, "What are you doing?"

This sent a shock wave through me that almost made me jump right out of my skin. I sat still, trying to gather my thoughts and determine my location and situation and evaluate the disaster area in front of me.

"You were asleep, weren't you?" Miriam asked. Now a bit more coherent, I realized what I had been doing. I had always been a chronic sleepwalker. The diet and the deprivation that came along with it was now causing me to sleep eat as well! Still, unsure whether this could be true, I asked, "Was I nibbling in my sleep?" "More like a six-course meal," said Miriam. We both sat and laughed for a good long time.

The next day Miriam packed up to leave. My problem had been solved by a lock on the refrigerator and a removal of all fattening foods in my house. Within twenty-four hours my diet mystery had been solved and I was on my way back to size 6!

## SURVIVAL HINTS

1. If your diet isn't working, there may be hidden problems that you can't see for yourself. If you've been dieting faithfully for more than three months and nothing is happening, consider working with a dieting coach, a nutritionist, or some other objective third party. Don't be afraid to ask for help.

2. Don't keep fattening foods around when you're dieting, or at any other time unless it's

absolutely unavoidable. These consist of those fabulous junk foods we all know and love, such as chips, dips, cookies, donuts, and other delightful but deadly snacks. Don't bring them into your house unless you lock them up and give someone else the key!

3. If you can't find a weight-guard, try a video camera equipped with a timer. You may find out all kinds of things that you don't expect, such as your cat prying open the fridge in the middle of the night for a tasty morsel!

# Dieting for Couch Potatoes

*Jack Mills*

I WAS A COUCH POTATO. I admit it. And I was starting to develop the shape of a potato: round top and bottom, columnar in the middle. Same sized chest, waist, and hips—or close to it. Talk about unibody construction. I was shaped like a gas pump!

Part of the problem was television. Having retired a few years earlier, I started indulging my taste for talk shows and soaps during the day, and then I had to watch all the sitcoms and cable shows at night.

But that was only part of the problem. Did you ever notice how many food commercials there are on television? Thirty-second spots, one after the other, bombard us with fast food ads for Wendy's, Burger King, White Castle, Mickey D's, Pizza Hut, Kentucky Fried, Popeye's, and all the others. And then there are the Mars and Snickers bars, Dunkin' Donuts and Krispy Kreme, Dairy Queen and Klondike, Häagen-Dazs and Ben & Jerry's. And what about the restaurant chains such as Olive Garden, Houlihan's, Friday's, Friendly's, and the rest?

One after another, these commercials show you delicious-looking, saliva-producing dishes, tempting foods you can almost taste and smell, all of which send you running for the refrigerator or the car keys or the telephone in desperate waves of sudden starvation! You'd think you had been living on bread and water, or grass and leaves for the intensity of those hunger pangs! And all this fattening food is everywhere, just waiting for you with open arms!

Being retired, I also stayed up very late at night, almost until dawn; sometimes I even watched infomercials, or else read the paper or a good murder mystery. I didn't have to get up for work, so why should I be disciplined at all? I'd earned a little self-indulgence, hadn't I, after all those years of hard work?

Still, little by little, I got bigger and bigger. By the time I was shopping at Big Man and living in sweats most of the time, my doctor threatened me with stomach stapling or a liquid diet because of my now sky-high blood pressure and cholesterol, not to mention obesity. I knew I had to take matters into my own hands—and fast.

I did some research, and here's what I discovered:

1. If you don't get enough sleep, you gain weight! I was stunned by this bit of news, and also delighted. I loved to sleep, but felt guilty sleeping past 7:00 a.m., and consequently was getting only about four hours sleep a night.

2. If you turn off the television for at least a few hours, you don't get as hungry because you don't have constant reminders of food flashing before your eyes.

3. If you walk even fifteen minutes a day, you can stop putting on weight. If you double that, you actually can start to lose a little.

4. If you find something to occupy your time, you won't be sitting around so much, and if you aren't bored, you won't turn to food for something to do.

With the wholehearted and somewhat disbelieving approval of my doctor, I bought a diet book and began to pay attention to portion control, calories and fats, and drinking more water. I began going to bed a few hours earlier, and slept for seven hours a night. Because I now felt better, I started going out more during the day.

Come September, I got a part-time job as a school crossing guard, and I really enjoyed being with the kids. All these changes got me off my fat butt, and the next thing I knew, I had to start wearing suspenders to hold up my pants!

Within six months, I'd almost effortlessly lost twenty-five pounds. My medical reports looked a lot better, and I was feeling great. Then I joined a bowling league at the insistence of my also-retired sister. Soon I was bowling three nights a week, had found a new group of friends, a social life, and a lot more to think about than television, food, and boredom.

That was ten years ago. I am now seventy years old and in great shape. I walk two miles every day, either outside or on my treadmill, and I've never been happier. I remarried a few years ago, and my wife is also a walker. We even take walking-tour vacations, and life is good.

So I guess if I hadn't had that brief flirtation with couch-potatohood, I might never have turned my life around. Sometimes, too much of a good thing really can turn out not to be so good after all!

## SURVIVAL HINTS

1. Go outside! If you are cooped up and inactive, you'll put on the pounds.
2. Turn to healthy social activities and hobbies that don't involve food and that make you more active in ways you enjoy, such as square dancing, ballroom dancing, or bowling.
3. If you're retired, consider getting a part-time job doing something you like; it will help keep you active and enjoying life.

# All or Nothing

*B. Lynn Goodwin*

I DREAD SHOPPING, so when I *had* to buy a new outfit, I started in familiar territory, the Encore
department at Nordstrom, where the large-size clothing is displayed. I skulked around, muttering and
shaking my head. "No, no, I don't think so."

A twenty-something sales clerk with a slightly thick
waistline and tightly braided hair stepped up. "Can I
help you?"

"I need something to wear to my nephew's wedding. It doesn't need to be dressy, and I don't know
what size I am anymore."

Tight Braids smiled or smirked; I didn't know
which. I surround myself with an emotional fortress

when I shop. "This department is for large-sized women. Nothing we have here would fit you."

"That's very nice to hear." My voice, soft and gentle, seemed to come from far away.

"Nothing we have here would fit you" is not a new phrase in my life, but I had never heard it used to suggest that I was too small. As a young girl, I was always at least twenty pounds over my ideal weight, and then, just as now, heavy teens were treated brutally in the mid-1960s. I had to wear what was appropriate for my shape, not the clothes that would have made me feel groovy or—shhh!—sexy. Personal preference in clothing styles meant nothing. All that mattered was what would fit and not look too bad.

When I tried out for a role in our senior play, *The Crucible,* I knew I couldn't be Abigail Williams or one of her cohorts: "You can't play a teenager. You're too fat. No one would believe you." The edict rang in my ears. Even though Arthur Miller described Mercy Lewis as a "fat, sly girl," I never got to read for the part.

Instead, I auditioned for Elizabeth Proctor, but Patti Thomas, who had a beautiful voice, won the role. I played an old woman, Rebecca Nurse. The message that I was too fat to be a teenager obscured the fact that Patti was better for the role. I was trapped by my compulsive consumption of M&Ms and my inability to break the cycle of dieting failures. I could see nothing else.

"You can't play a teenager unless you lose weight."

"If you want to have friends, lose weight."

"If you want dates, lose weight."

I internalized the concept that fat people could not have a life; consequently, I let go of my dreams. Proms and parties slid away. If I wanted them badly enough, I was told, I would stay on my diet, but diets lasted three days before gnawing hunger overcame my resolve. In those days I believed that a magic secret, reserved for others, eluded me. The failures stacked up.

When I was in my twenties, I started a diet every morning. I drank coffee for breakfast and ate lettuce with low-cal dressing for lunch. I supplemented this fare with chips and candy from the vending machines. As a dedicated high school teacher, I worked harder than most and deserved a treat, so I nibbled in my car, nibbled while I cooked, and munched my way through my work: correcting adolescents' essays and planning the next day's lessons.

By my mid-thirties, I was still a high school teacher but I was also teaching drama at community colleges. I ate in my car between schools. One night after rehearsal at one college, I stopped to buy groceries. As I drove home on the freeway, I started melting frozen pasta, piece by piece, on my tongue. Though my tongue was numb when I got home, I ate Pepperidge Farm Goldfish while I nuked a Lean Cuisine, then munched my way through cookies and ice cream in my efforts to anesthetize the day's frustrations.

When I was in my forties, my metabolism slowed down, and I stopped looking in the mirror. I could not bear to see the fat, miserable creature looking back.

One day after my teaching career and a six-year stint of caring for my aging mother had ended, I took my life back. I read a weight-loss flyer and found a comfortable fit with a therapist in Berkeley. She offered no diet. Instead, we discussed my eating habits, and she suggested changes. I did not get on her scale. Knowing that I would check in each week kept me eating safe foods.

My therapist didn't judge me or smother me with expectations. She told me that my clothes were getting looser and that I was looking thinner. She supported me as we talked about events that had triggered my eating.

Months went by. One day at work, a colleague looked me over and said, "You look different. Have you been sick?"

"No."

"You look thinner. Your face is thinner."

"I've been losing weight for almost a year." I could feel myself beaming.

"Really? How are you doing it?"

"I don't buy boxes of crackers or cookies anymore." I had quit the chocolate chip cookies and salty crackers cold turkey. I was on the all-or-nothing plan where junk food was concerned, and I chose nothing. I no longer stopped at McDonald's. When I arrived home without having stuffed my face on the way, I felt good enough to go walking. I gave up donuts and chips and stopped my daily visits to the convenience store. I bought broccoli, apples, and mushrooms for snacks.

"How much have you lost?" she asked.

How I dreaded that question. The scale's fluctuating numbers complicated everything and brought on bingeing and guilt. "Around forty pounds," I guessed. There was a great deal to be said for keeping it simple.

The mirror is my measuring stick now, along with glimpses of myself reflected in store windows. When I bloat up, I know the feeling will subside if I stay out of the kitchen for a few hours. I've begun to accept that weight-loss is a process of ups and downs, just like life. When the weight creeps back on, I turn it around before it gets out of control.

Why do these new habits stick with me season after season? Is it because I admitted out loud that I was addicted to Entenmann's chocolate chip cookies, unable

to live without my drug of choice? Did they stay because I learned I could eat a bit too much one day and
make up for it the next? Or did they last because I admitted there were holes in my life that food could
never fill?

Part of me knows the weight will be back if I don't
face the emotions that trigger my eating, and that
nudges me to explore my feelings as I did the day my
therapist asked, "What did you wear to your nephew's
wedding?"

I sighed. "A loose knit sweater, kind of soft and
delicate."

She waited, her head cocked slightly, her eyes ex-
pectant.

"It goes with a rayon crepe skirt that has rich tropical palm leaves on a dark background and a flaring
ruffle that swishes when I walk." I felt a broad smile,
despite my guarded tone. I loved the swish of that
ruffle.

"Montana can be cold at the beginning of May. Did
you take a jacket?"

"My sister said I should, but I wasn't about to go
shopping again, so I found a black one that my
mother gave me years ago. It never did fit me, and the
tags were still on it. I knew it would look perfect with
the skirt, but I had felt like a stuffed sausage en-
shrouded in black casing the last time I had it on. This

time, though, I put my arms in the sleeves and pulled it on without tugging."

My stomach quaked. My therapist looked at me with the tiniest smile at the corners of her mouth.

"I guess I should have known it would fit, but it surprised me. I was so proud, and I felt the most amazing smile radiating across my face."

My voice caught. I stopped for a moment. My therapist said nothing.

"I put on the whole outfit and stood in front of a mirror that once hung in my father's apartment."

I stopped again. Would my parents be proud if they could see me now, or would they wonder why I had not lost the weight while they were still here to see it? I was afraid I would cry if I asked that question out loud, so I took another deep breath and went on:

"I was a short middle-aged woman, larger than some, but smaller than many, a work in progress, no longer the old teenaged wannabe."

"And how did that make you feel?" the therapist asked.

"Happy. Maybe that was the real goal all along."

She smiled. "Maybe so."

Our time was up and she walked me to the door. Out on the street, I did not even think of rewarding myself with a cookie.

## SURVIVAL HINTS

1. Try to determine what emotional triggers may be causing you to overeat, and then work out ways to deal with them and to substitute a different response besides eating.

2. Don't use food as solace when something is bothering you; instead, try to deal more directly with the issue. It'll help save inches from piling onto your body, and you'll be happier in the long run.

3. If you need help, seek out a qualified therapist who deals with weight-loss issues. And remember, you aren't alone—many people need a bit of extra help when weight gain has emotional roots, so don't be afraid to ask for help.

B. Lynn Goodwin is the editor of WriterAdvice, http://www.writeradvice.com, and she contributes author interviews and book reviews to the Web site. She writes book reviews for the *Small Press Review* and Web site reviews for the California Writers Club, has been published in the *Oakland Tribune* and the *Contra Costa Times,* and has a piece titled "Needed" in the winter issue of *Flashquake.*

# There Really Is
# Such a Thing as *Too* Thin

*Richard Pendrake*

MANY DIETERS LOOK AT thin people with resentment. I've heard the suspicions: "That person looks anorexic," "Look! a human coat-hanger," or even "I bet that person has a grape for lunch and supper." Although eating disorders can cause people to lose weight in unhealthy ways, I do not have the problem of trying to lose weight in harmful ways. I have a problem trying to keep weight on. This is still a dieter's story.

"A problem? How can that be a problem?" asks my friend, who is eyeing my second lunch entrée and slice of cake for dessert. He knows I don't have a disease and that I am not undergoing treatment that would cause me to lose weight. It must seem impossible for a person to have a problem trying to keep weight on.

After some erratic behavior in my youth and some dramatic mood swings, my doctor diagnosed me with the not-rare-enough condition of hypoglycemia: low blood sugar. Though I haven't had a thorough review of the root cause of this problem, I link it with my high metabolism. I simply cannot put on weight.

Let's go back to the lunch in question. It is a business lunch. My friend, we'll call him David, is exercising regularly in an effort to lose a few pounds. He's looking at the chocolate cake on the menu with a desire usually reserved for his girlfriend when he picks her up for a date. Now that he's dieting, the cake looks better in proportion to its inaccessibility.

"Why don't you eat it," he asks, hoping to enjoy it vicariously.

"Just because I'm going to be hungry in an hour doesn't mean I can eat a lot now," I gripe. I realize it's a gripe, but it's a common misunderstanding. The inability to gain weight doesn't come with a license to eat as much as I want whenever I want. My appetite ranges from generous at times to meager at others. Still, I know I will be hungry in an hour, no matter what I eat. Being thin chains me to food.

"Just a slice of cake," he continues, drooling. "Dessert."

A thing about hypoglycemia: Natural sugars do better than dessert sugars, but that's not saying much. The small ham sandwich I ate for lunch was good, and it raised my blood sugar level. The potato chips provided me a short-term boost with the consequence of later causing my blood sugar to drop quickly. I chose water to drink not because I want to keep my slim figure but because the sugars in tea or cola would be destructive. So would the chocolate cake's frosting.

Instead of my blood sugar leveling off slowly over time, if I eat or drink too much sugar, my blood sugar declines rapidly, no matter where I am. So if my boss calls an impromptu meeting or if a problem occurs at work that I must respond to, my blood sugar will not listen. I simply cannot eat the cake for fear of the possible consequences.

"Look," I explain, "I have hypoglycemia, and I need to watch what I eat so that I can keep my blood sugar stable." Ears perk up around the table.

I listen to the standard suggestions. Eat red meat; don't eat red meat; eat starches; don't eat starches; try lots of veggies; veggies won't help you. In the end, the conflicting advice is not very helpful to a person with such a condition and a fast metabolism. Rather than consider all these well-meaning suggestions, I accept my responsibility and identify the foods I eat by keeping a journal; this helps me over time to achieve my goals: feeling good and keeping my weight on rather than off.

A woman who is trying to lose a significant amount of weight stares at me blankly: "You mean neither of us can have dessert today?"

Yes. Thin people as well as dieters should not eat dessert or load their plates with just any kind of food. People should exercise within the limits prescribed by their doctors, no matter what their weight. Why do you think so many thin people go to gyms? Whether one is too fat or too thin, there is no magic pill to solve the problem. Unless the treatment is sensible, it simply replaces one problem with another.

I don't want to tell my coworkers what I am about to admit: I resent people who can gain weight. Being skinny does not help a body image all the time. I get unwanted attention at lunch as the person who theoretically could eat anything on the menu. And the weight I don't have helps others develop the defined muscles that look so appealing on people who exercise correctly.

The friend who wants to shed a few pounds and the woman who wishes to revert to her college weight could very well have an advantage over me. They might have an end-point for their objectives. Maybe they put on the pounds in a short-term period of eating and drinking too much instead of battling it throughout their lives. Although some people have difficulty losing weight because they have slow metabolisms, I suspect that some dieters are simply trying to lose weight because they think they have to. "Give it to me," I've joked before, wishing such a fat transfusion actually could take place. These are people who are healthy and have not a pound more or less than they probably should have at that moment. If one hundred reasonable adults were polled, they would all probably say they needed to lose weight.

For those people, I would offer the following advice: Don't judge me as someone who is thin by choice, and I won't judge you as someone who enjoys being able to eat the foods I want to eat. A lot of people face personal dieting challenges, no matter what their weight. Some diets end when a certain weight is achieved; but, for most of us, the trick is to find what is personally healthy and to stick with those healthy activities that can help maintain the desired weight.

And that chocolate cake you're eyeing? When we're both in shape, we can have a slice together.

# SURVIVAL HINTS

1. Whether you want to gain weight or lose it, eat meals and snacks that promote good health. Excessive amounts of sugar and fat will not make you feel better and can have long-term negative effects on everyone's health, even that of thin people!

2. Keep a food diary or journal to help you determine what works best for your particular weight program. You may find some unexpected surprises, not to mention triggers that cause allergic reactions. You could also become aware of other pitfalls caused by specific foods.

# A Work in Process

*Barbara A. Craig*

I AM A WORK IN PROCESS. I do not want to say that I am trying to get into shape. I have a shape. My shape is larger than I want it to be, but it is a shape. For years, I have been attempting to become smaller, but I keep adding to my shape. This has to change. I have been told that you receive according to the type of energy you put out. If you emit negative energy, you attract negativity. So I have been laboring to get into shape, and my shape has obeyed.

I know that my attitude is not the cause of my excess bulk, but I need the right mindset to achieve my goals. Part of my weight gain was caused by stress eating and another part by my heart defect. Without going into too much detail, my heart works twice as hard as a normal heart at rest. What this means is that I can very easily get sick. If I have the beginnings of a cold and I continue to exercise, I cannot fight the cold and I end up with bronchitis. So I cannot work out as much as I would like.

This problem is a cruel joke. My metabolism works only if I exercise. No matter what I do, if I do not exercise, I will gain weight. Even if I follow a perfect diet, I gain weight. There was a time when I did not exercise for a long time because I was afraid of dying. I almost fainted in a step-bench class, and from that time on all exercise stopped. I now realize that there are other forms of exercise besides high-impact aerobics. I have found that my heart can tolerate belly dancing, Pilates, yoga, and stability ball.

Weight loss is a battle I must win mentally before lasting changes can be made. I am taking a new approach this time. I am looking at weight loss as a lifelong process. It is harder for me to give up if I am working within a process.

So phase one—exercise—of my new life process is going well. If I am not up to exercising one day, I try to exercise the next day. I used to get discouraged and give up quickly. I used to believe that if I did not work out for an hour or two at once, the exercise did not count. I also believed that if I did not increase the length of my workout every week, exercising would no longer be effective. So I would start off well, and then by the end of two months, I would say, "I don't have time or energy to exercise for three hours a day; what's the point?" I will not let myself fall into this trap of self-sabotage again. I am taking my exercise in smaller bites. Forty minutes in the morning, then shorter programs after work, usually from ten to thirty minutes. My goal is now more reasonable: four or five hours a week.

Phase one of my process—exercise—feeds phase two—eating healthy. One word I hate is "diet." I think that the definition should be changed. If I had my way, the dictionary definition would tell the truth: Diet v. 1. To cause extreme self-suffering; 2. To follow the latest food craze; 3. To lose a few pounds and gain back twice as many.

My mindset changes when I say I am on a diet. This is what happens: All food starts to look good. Even foods I have never even liked. Then I become obsessed with not eating foods I always hated to begin with.

When dieting, it has been said that if you deprive yourself of any one food, you will eventually go insane and proceed to eat your way through the snack isle at the closest convenience store. I do not want that to

happen. So if I am in the diet mindset and I see something I usually do not like, I still feel deprived, so I eat
the nasty morsel. Then I am proud of myself for not
eating more. Therefore I resolve never to diet again
because thinking about "dieting" does not work for
me. Instead, I embark on a new way of thinking about
how and what I eat.

Phase two consists of portion control and better
food choices. This part is like walking a tightrope.
When I am exercising, I tend to ask, "How many
Pilates one-hundreds will I have to do to work off that
peanut butter cup?" So right away I am doing better.

But what I am afraid of is rationalization and PMS.
They are the monkey wrenches of my weight-loss
process. I am afraid that if I start to overdo process
one, exercising, I can justify eating poorly in process
two. I do not want to rationalize when I eat a pizza because I have already burned off the calories and fat in
the pizza. To fight this, I have picked out a couple of
dresses I cannot buy until I lose weight. I am hoping
that the dress craving will kill the pizza craving.

I have read a diet book written by a well-known and
popular television doctor. This is a great guideline and
motivation for my process. But one point really scares
me. The doctor says that you can actually gain weight
by looking at food. How scary is that? Looking at food
can trigger a hormone that slows your metabolism! I

love to cook; I used to love watching the food channel on television. Now, I watch the fitness channel. If you can gain weight by watching food, maybe I can lose weight by watching exercise. After all, that would only be fair.

I am not on a diet. I cannot acquire a different body type than the one I already have. And I am a work in process. I have been a work in process for a little over a month now. I have not weighed myself, otherwise I would have results to report, but I have noticed changes in how my clothes fit.

Rather than dieting to change my weight, I am changing my life, my habits, and my mindset in my quest to become healthy. Results will take time; I am and will be okay with that. I will build my life around this process and I will succeed!

## SURVIVAL HINTS

1. Consult your doctor before you begin a diet. You can seriously damage your health by undertaking a diet that isn't appropriate for you. Even if you are in perfect health, you should follow a medically approved diet or you could damage your health by using a plan that isn't scientifically proven to be safe.

2.  Attitude is very important when you are trying to lose weight. If you adjust your mindset to realistic goals, you have a much better chance of attaining them and maintaining your new weight and size after you achieve those goals.

3.  It's important to work with what you have, rather than try to be like anyone else. Self-acceptance is important in achieving dieting goals, so be sure to measure yourself only against yourself, rather than against someone whose body is totally different. Remember, we don't all have to look like supermodels to be beautiful, and such standards are both fleeting and changeable!

# 8

# When Your Diet Drives Everyone Else Crazy

### Dieting's for the Dogs
Evelyn M. Fazio

### He Said, She Said
Edward Stevens

### The Dieting Vegetarians
Maria Ross

# Sanity Quiz

You've been on your diet for three weeks, and friends and family are going crazy because of it. Not only are you watching everything you eat, but everything *they* put in *their* mouths. You insist that they not serve bread, butter, or pasta at any meal you attend, and you can't stop lecturing them about the benefits of your diet. You are in danger of becoming a pariah with no friends left.

Do you

A. zip your lips and stop talking about dieting
B. invite them over to dinner—but use your diet principles when cooking the meal
C. tolerate their disdain
D. give up and rejoin the ranks of the sane

If you answered yes to any of these questions, then you're probably driving someone crazy with your diet. Read on and see how some of us have coped with this quandary.

# Dieting's for the Dogs

*Evelyn M. Fazio*

I'VE HEARD IT SAID that people have a hard time going on diets and sticking to them. But does anyone ever think about the innocent bystanders who also have to put up with them?

First of all, they're crabby. So right away there's trouble. Even though you might normally be allowed to nap on the nice velvet sofa, when your human is dieting, look out! I never saw so many rolled-up newspapers coming my way in my life!

Second of all, there are no table scraps. And if there were, *they'd* be eating them, not you. It's really bad. You can sit there looking soulfully into your master's eyes, drooling with the best of them, and nothing happens! You could die of hunger. And table scraps are the only real food you get, especially when you consider that you can't count the disgusting canned stuff they give you, or that horrible dry kibble—you could choke to death, and we never really chew anything anyway!

Third of all, they're really distracted. Probably because they're hungry—and you can relate to that! So they forget to feed you at the regular time, and they forget to take you out for a walk until you practically climb over their heads and dance around with your legs crossed trying not to have an accident. It's not easy.

So how do you survive? Well, there's water. If they remember to fill your bowl. Water helps fill you up and gets rid of the hunger pangs for a while. My human also was saying to her husband that water is supposed to flush out all the fat you're burning off. They should give me that fat—it's the best part of a meal!

The next survival technique is to run around a lot, with or without barking. Running keeps your metabolism up, and it will distract you from thinking about food. My human said that when she exercises, it takes the edge off her hunger, especially if she does it before a meal.

Another great weight-loss technique that humans are just figuring out is sleep. You have to get enough sleep to lose weight. It's really important, and something we canines have known about for a really long time.

Another bit of advice is do not overeat. You know what happens to us dogs—we eat really fast, run around like lunatics, barking and leaping as if we had stepped on thumbtacks—and then, watch out—we start horking up our entire dinner!

I always hear my human talking about portion control, and it applies to us, too. She also uses smaller plates to make the meal look larger. She used this tactic on the cat—not that he doesn't deserve it, mind you. She took one of those little saucers from the espresso cups and fed him his dinner on it! I don't think it fooled him one bit. We animals are a lot smarter than those humans—they think their big brains mean something, but we all know it's mostly wasted space!

My last bit of advice is to be patient with your humans. They will probably be a trial until they're done with their diets, but they'll be so happy when it's over that they'll probably celebrate with food! So stick around—with their shrunken stomachs, there's bound to be a lot more left for you.

## SURVIVAL HINTS

1. Try to keep your mind off food as much as possible by finding things to do, such as grooming your dog, playing with your cat, washing the car, cleaning out a closet—anything but eating or being near food.

2. Try to be as active as you can, even if it means walking upstairs instead of taking the elevator, walking the dog a few extra times a day, and parking a healthy distance from your door, the store, and your office.

3. Drink lots of water. We've said it before, and we can't say it enough. It'll fill you up. And make sure you keep your animals' water bowls full, too! They will appreciate it more than you realize.

4. Don't watch television. In the average half-hour show, there are literally dozens of food commercials that will show nothing but mouth-watering things that can derail you in two seconds flat. Watch movies on DVDs instead; you will be able to control what you're exposed to. If all else fails, read a book and improve your mind at the same time. There are no food commercials in them!

5. Use smaller plates to control portions and make them appear larger. So much of appetite has to

do with perception. If you perceive that you have a larger portion than the one actually on your plate, you will not feel deprived.

6. Get plenty of sleep! It's been proven that a minimum of seven to eight hours of sleep helps you lose weight. Now isn't that the best news you've ever heard? But naps don't count—it all has to happen during your nights' sleep to work properly. Give it a try.

# He Said, She Said

*Edward Stevens*

"I'M ON A DIET," she said. "Well, I'm not," I said to
Ellen, my wife of fifteen dieting years. We have had
this argument several times during our life together.
But for some reason, this time I was the one who was
suffering yet again on *her* diet.

Ellen had to try every diet she heard about.
Whether it be in a book, a magazine, or just hearsay, if
someone, anyone, said it worked, she had to try it.
Now Ellen is not overweight; maybe she could shed a
few pounds, but by no means is it a must. What's a little more in the caboose? Just a little more to hold
onto, I say!

She was simply addicted to dieting and torturing me was par for the course.

Whenever she decided she looked too fat in a dress, a skirt, a shirt, or even a glove, it was time to set off into dieting hell. Most people only torture *themselves* while dieting, but Ellen insisted upon using me as her support system. I don't remember promising to love, honor and diet together when I took my wedding vows. But somewhere in her *fat* mind, she had convinced herself that if she had to go through it, then so would I.

"What's for dinner?" I squeaked out while walking through the kitchen. Ellen turned around. She looked like the possessed girl in *The Exorcist.* "*ASSsssparagus* and spinach, you know it's Friday, don't you?" I think saliva was running out of the corner of her mouth when I now, scared, but standing my ground, said, "What is it, Good Friday? Where's the beef?"

Beef was Ellen's weakness and I knew it. She loved a good steak. An eye for an eye round was my motto. If she can torture me, I can torture her. "What did you just say?" was the black-eyed hissing-hell creature's reply. "I said, 'Where's the beef?'" I replied, as I braced myself against the counter for incoming flying objects. "You want beef? You know I am on a diet and can't have meat. So now you are going to torture me and eat my favorite food in front of me while I sit here and suffer?"

"Who the hell wanted to go on this diet, anyway?" I shot back.

Noticing the look of failure on Ellen's face, I retreated. "Look," I said, "I can suffer through another veggie-only night if you will give up this constant insanity of thinking you're overweight. Your caboose may be loose but it is as fine as the day I married you, if not better." Ellen only smiled and did not reply.

But that night I ate the best steak of my life, followed by a dessert that I never thought Ellen had in her, even after fifteen years!

# The Dieting Vegetarians

*Maria Ross*

NOTHING WILL DRIVE you crazier than cooking for a vegetarian when you aren't one yourself. Nothing! Oh, yes, there is one thing. Cooking for vegetarians on a diet is even worse, especially if you have no experience with this group of dieters.

About twenty years ago, I became friends with several vegetarians. Some were vegetarian for ethical reasons, some because of health concerns, and some because of their religious convictions. It didn't matter. All I knew was that I was a carnivore, and was used to cooking with meat. Most of my culinary repertoire then centered on chicken, and those recipes that didn't involved various permutations of pasta with meat sauce.

One day, two of my strict vegetarian friends were coming to dinner; not only did they not eat meat but they were both on diets. It was a double whammy for this chef!

I wracked my brains about what to feed them. I had to skip chicken and fish, and the lasagna that I was in the mood for was probably out, too, considering the ground beef and meat sauce, not to mention the high fat content of the ricotta and mozzarella. So I'd be serving salad. But what could I find to go with it?

I went to the supermarket and trawled the dairy aisle, wondering what to do. And then I spotted them! Low-fat ricotta and low-fat mozzarella. A dream come true. Now all I had to do was concoct a batch of red sauce—minus the meat. Who knew what *that* would taste like? But I was determined.

Back home with my purchases, which included a big basket of ripe plum tomatoes, I got busy chopping and working with the blender to perfect a smooth, sweet batch of sauce. I sautéed onions and garlic and stirred in the raw tomato sauce. I added a little of this and a little of that, some fresh oregano, some fresh basil, and it tasted . . . flat. What was I going to do?

After pondering the contents of the refrigerator for a few seconds, I spied the jar of freshly grated romano cheese. I stirred some in, waited a bit, and tasted—that did it. Now it tasted like food!

As I quickly assembled a big tray of lasagna, I was careful to hold back on the amount of ricotta between the layers, as well as the thickness of the mozzarella on top. I was sure that by restraining myself in this way, I was further cutting down on the amount of fat and calories that I'd be serving my dieting guests. I then popped the dish into the oven and prepared some steamed asparagus as a side dish. I decided to squeeze a bit of lemon over the spears for flavor, without adding any extra calories or fat. I complimented myself on my efforts.

The guests arrived an hour later, and soon we all sat down to dinner. My father, in town for the weekend, was a committed carnivore and had been teasing me all day about this meatless meal he was being forced to share.

Everyone took a generous helping of the salad, which was dressed with a dribble of olive oil and a splash of vinegar, and a serving of the main dish— smaller portions for the dieters, of course. And then Dad, with a mischievous gleam in his eye, intoned, "Something's missing!" We all started to laugh.

I held my breath while the vegetarians took a bite. Dead silence. Then, "Mm-mmm-mmm! This is wonderful!" I began to breathe normally, the color returned to my cheeks, and I watched, wide-eyed, as they inhaled their portions. Looking longingly at the delicious contents of the baking dish, they both said they'd better stop now or they'd finish off the entire batch. I was thrilled, and I relaxed for the rest of the meal.

My vegetarians were so delighted with the lasagna that they took home some leftovers, and I began to see that it was indeed possible to survive cooking and eating the vegetarian way without giving up flavor. And wouldn't you know it, only five years later, I joined their ranks myself!

## SURVIVAL HINTS

1. Try to find ways of cutting out excess fat and calories, because both matter. Use low-fat ingredients wherever possible, and avoid synthetic ingredients.

2. Portion size is very important when feeding dieters. Either start out with a small serving, or else let them serve themselves. This is even better—it avoids any type of implied judgment on your part.

3. Don't be afraid to tackle new ways of eating— you might just end up joining the other team!

# 9

# When You Have Dieting Helpers

*Next Window, Please*
Alyssia Ruiz

*Body Inventory*
Amanda Samson

# Sanity Quiz

There is always someone looking to help even when it comes to *your* diet. This time, it's your best friend, Susie. Susie has never had an ounce of fat on her in her life. She is a human stick. Although Susie is skinny, she always feels the need to help you on your weight-loss quest. Today, Susie has taken it upon herself to enroll you in an Overeaters' Anonymous group.

Do you

A. thank Susie for her support
B. tell her thanks, but no thanks
C. tell her she knows nothing about how you feel and that she should mind her own business
D. go to the meetings even though you don't want to—so that Susie doesn't find out you hated her so-called gift

If you answered yes to any of these questions, you know someone like Suzie, or have had to deal with dieting helpers. Rather than let your frustrations send you to Ben & Jerry's for solace, read on and discover some better ways to cope.

# Next Window, Please

*Alyssia Ruiz*

"WOULD YOU LIKE TO place an order?" the pimple-coated kid said to me as I drove up to the McDonald's window. "Yes," I said. "I would like a *Big* Mac, a *biggie-*size fry, and, um, I guess a *diet* coke." I added, "You see, I'm on a diet."

The little blister looked at me as if I was out of my mind. Having quite the view from his window perch, his glance swept over my 250-pound figure like a razor cutting through a cardboard box. "Whatever, lady," he replied.

Now I could have come back with something equally hurtful, such as running to the drugstore and buying a tube of acne cream to deliver through his drive-thru window. But the kid was right. Who am I kidding? A diet soda on top of this calorie mountain? It was ridiculous. That day, I cried over my Big Mac, the whole time I was eating it, in fact. I knew something had to be done to stop this insanity. But what? Was there really a way to shed the pounds I had gained over a five-year period quickly enough to make me achieve my goal before I gave up? I had my doubts.

I spent the next afternoon at the bookstore looking for the magic fix that would spell out the entire plan for me. Well, I don't know whether you have ever tried going to the bookstore for a diet book, but I discovered that there are dozens to choose from. Too many, and all claiming to be like no other, the super fix. As I sat trying to figure out which one to purchase, I saw a bright yellow one on the bottom shelf. Then, just as I bent for it, I was bumped from behind, literally on my behind. Irate, I stood up and came face to face with that same boy, the fast-food Pimplestiltskin.

Now I was really angry. Not only had this kid insulted me about my weight problem but he had caused me to bump my head on the bookshelf, leaving an egg-shaped knob in the dead center of my forehead.

"Why don't you watch where you're going?" I said. "Why don't you watch where you put that thing?" he replied. That was it for me. Now I was furious. "I think you are in the wrong section," I shot back. "The books on leprosy are in the next section."

A moment of silence overcame us both while we stood still just staring into each other's eyes. Suddenly, we broke into hysterical laughter. The realization of what we were doing had hit us both at the same moment. We were torturing each other because of our own shortcomings.

That day, Pimplestiltskin and I became friends and we hope our friendship will last forever. I have lost twenty-eight pounds by buying salad for lunch at his window, and he now has the clearest skin I have ever seen thanks to my suggestions about acne medication. And now I call him by his real name, Jared.

## SURVIVAL HINTS

1. Sometimes a comment from a stranger can really hurt, but it also might be the only time you hear the truth, so pay attention.
2. Don't be afraid to reach out for help; remember that it can come from the place you least expect it. And you never know, you just might find a new friend at the same time.
3. If you want to select a diet book, try to get a recommendation from someone who's used one successfully, or read reviews online or in newspapers or magazines. There really are too many to choose from without help!

# Body Inventory

*Amanda Samson*

"I CAN'T STAND the way I look," I said. "What's the matter with you? You look good to me," he said, with those "why don't we go in the other room" eyes. But sex was the last thing on my mind. I couldn't stand looking at myself, let alone having someone else look at me.

"My arms are fat, my rear is huge, and my legs look like they're Jell-O-filled. Where the hell did my body go?" "We had three kids, you know," he replied. "Oh, and that's supposed to make me feel better? So you do agree that I'm fat." He didn't know what to say without sticking his foot any farther into his mouth. He was already knee-deep and he wanted to retreat.

"So you gained a few pounds," he replied. "I gained way more than a few, and I've been on this stupid diet for more than six months!" I belted back. "And look at me. Nothing, I've gotten nowhere." "You have so," he said, and stomped out of the room.

I stood in front of the mirror and stared at the alien who had taken over my body and inflated it to this gargantuan size. Then I began to cry. What was all this effort about if I wasn't getting anywhere? Why was I restricting what I ate if it wasn't helping? I ran to the kitchen and grabbed the box of donuts; one by one, I shoved them in. I had three in my stomach and was working on number four when my husband entered the room carrying the small journal I started when I began my diet. I hadn't written anything in well over a month.

He said, "Get on the scale." I did. He took the pen and noted my weight, along with the date. Then, after flipping back twenty pages, he handed me the journal.

I was ten pounds lighter on today's page than I had been twenty pages back! I *was* making progress. It was slow, but it was there in black and white. So all the effort had been rewarded. My husband knew the diet was working for me even though I didn't. I guess sometimes you just need another opinion!

# SURVIVAL HINTS

1. Don't be too hard on yourself. Self-discipline, not criticism, will help you stick to your diet. Beating yourself up only makes you feel worse, and it might make you give up your diet efforts entirely.

2. Don't give up, because slower weight loss is safer than crash dieting, and it leads to permanent lifestyle changes for the better.

3. It helps to keep a written inventory of your weight if you have a lot to lose; you may be losing more and doing better than you realize.

4. Sometimes it helps to have positive reinforcement from someone other than yourself; it's difficult to be objective about oneself most of the time, and even more so when you are dieting.

# 10

# When Your Diet Is
# Frustrating You

# Sanity Quiz

Its 6:00 p.m. on Monday. You have just come home from a long day at work only to find, to your surprise, that your husband and kids have pulled together and, in a group effort, made dinner for you. You have been on a diet for three weeks—one where you must measure and weigh everything you eat. Unfortunately, they have prepared extra crispy fried chicken, your favorite meal and biggest weakness.

Do you

A. thank them all for the effort but decline
B. eat it anyway for the kid's sake and use that as an excuse to overeat
C. yell at your husband for sabotaging your diet and tempting you
D. pile your plate high, and, when no one is looking, slip half to the dog
E. throw the fit to end all fits

If you answered yes to even one of these questions, you need to read on and find out how your fellow dieters got around this type of situation.

# The Joys of Dieting

*J. Alesandro*

OH, THE JOYS OF DIETING. Let's see—there's starving yourself, eating foods you dislike, weighing in at every chance you get to see whether, by some miracle, you have actually lost an ounce or two. There is your growling stomach, too.

That reminds me of a story. I have been on a diet for more than two years now. But when I first started, it was really difficult. I was way overweight and used to consuming whatever I wanted. But then my doctor told me that if I didn't cut down, I would be risking my life. That day, my wife decided it was her new mission to make me healthy. So she got rid of all the goodies in the house and set out to make me fit as a fiddle.

After about three weeks of torture, as a reward and surprise, she took me out to my favorite restaurant. It was a busy night and we had to wait to get in. Since I had been on this diet, my stomach had become very vocal by way of reminding me at every opportunity that I was starving it to death.

I'd say there were probably about twenty people in line that night and we were at the tail end. All of a sudden, my stomach let out a cry for help sharp enough to pierce a hole in a tin can. All the chattering in the line abruptly stopped. As people stood around listening and looking for the source, they again began to chatter and giggle, but this time it was about the mysterious noise. Knowing full well where it came from, my wife said, "Was that you?"

I hung my head, leaned in close to her, and said, "It wasn't me—it's the one you are starving to death." Again, a noise louder than before screeched from my stomach. This time, everyone in line turned and looked at me. It was unmistakable. I was the source of the noise. Just then, the hostess came to the podium to call for the next party whose table was ready. She said, "Who is next?" Without hesitation, the couple in the front and then everyone else in line turned around and pointed to me!

## SURVIVAL HINTS

1. Eat when you are hungry to avoid bingeing, but don't use hunger as an excuse to binge.

2. Don't starve yourself—it won't work, and it will make you more likely to cheat, eat the wrong foods, and overeat; starving yourself will also make you crabby because your blood sugar will drop to the danger zone.

3. If you want to get a table quickly in a restaurant, make sure the hostess hears your stomach growling. It may not work every time, but it sure did for this writer!

# Maybe

*Toni Scott*

"ONE, TWO, one two, oh screw it. I've exercised enough." One, two, or maybe three Tastycakes later, I'm satisfied. Maybe the perfect diet only involves working off the calories of the "extra" food you eat every day.

Maybe if they wouldn't make the fattening food so damned tasty to begin with, we wouldn't be in this situation in the first place.

Maybe the scale has a problem detecting your correct weight and is adding pounds that don't belong to you or they are left over from the last fat blimp who stepped on it.

Maybe your jeans shrank in the dryer and it's not your butt that's getting bigger but it's your jeans that are getting smaller.

Maybe if I had been born of French descent and not a fat-ass cupcake-eating American, I would be sleek and sexy, not fat and frumpy.

Maybe it's time to sit back and look at ourselves, because for many of us, weight is in the top ten list of our issues. And maybe there is no one to blame but ourselves.

Nobody forced you to eat a second helping. Nobody shoved that cake down your throat. Nobody told you to super-size every meal you consume.

Maybe we are always on the run. Maybe we starve ourselves and then gorge. Maybe we become addicted to processed foods and crave them like a junkie. Maybe we live for convenience, but convenience is fattening. And maybe fattening turns into maddening, and maybe now you have to remove all that you have put in.

Maybe now it's time for that diet; oh, so many to choose from. Where, oh, where shall I begin?

Maybe I'll just eat one instead of two. And maybe I will adjust three reps to four.

Maybe I will move to France, and maybe I will stick to a plan. Maybe I will start today, and maybe I will finally find a way to lose that weight at last!

# SURVIVAL HINTS

1. Do what works for you, and don't worry if it's a bit unconventional. Original approaches to weight loss can work better than what everyone else does.

2. Be forgiving of yourself if you slip up on your diet. Don't use a small slip-up as an excuse to binge; this is a common pitfall for many dieters after the smallest dieting transgression. Just move forward and get back on your diet program. In the long run, a small mistake won't make much difference, and you can always do a few extra laps in the pool, or trips around the block, or an extra bit of time on the treadmill if it'll make you feel better about your small mistake.

3. And remember, you're only human; you don't have to be perfect, just determined and realistic to reach your weight-loss goals.

# Secret Diets

*Natasha Forbes*

WHAT IS IT ABOUT DIETS that really make you go stir-crazy? If you go on a fruit-only diet, the vegetables you never ate before suddenly become must-haves. If you go on a vegetables-only diet, the fruit you have never before craved suddenly becomes irresistible. When we're dieting, why is it we always want what we can't have, or usually never even want?

I compulsively try new diet plans. If it's new and claims to work, you can be damn sure I'm gonna try it. Maybe just to test it; hell, I have been proving diet experts wrong for years—what's one more on my list? I'm game. What's another week or two of sheer torture, mood altering, sacrificial, save-yourself-before-you-jump torment? Even if you lose only a pound or two, it's worth it. A pound can mean being condemned to wearing the size 12 Levis you wore right after giving birth to your third child. You know, the ones you were going to throw out because you swore up and down that you weren't having any more kids and *never* were going to be that big again? But two years of taking care of and cooking for three kids have taken their toll on your shape.

Whether it is in your butt, thighs, or belly, you are suddenly able to see the cookie-eating, cupcake-toting results from the monster within. Your size 8 is still in the closet calling your name, but your size 12 butt can't hear it through all the fat!

Sometimes the worst thing you can possibly do while on a diet is to tell someone you live with that you are dieting. Why? Because then every time your partner or a family member looks at you while you are eating, you will worry about what he or she is thinking rather than concentrate on reaching your goal: losing weight.

This only leads to a new and hidden source of eating: closet eating. You can actually become fatter just because you have made someone else aware of your problem. That's because when you make someone aware of your diet, that person not only treats you differently but also looks at you differently. Your eating patterns are being watched to see whether they have changed and your shape is studied to see whether it has changed. Telling your husband is, in my opinion, the biggest mistake of all.

Look, if you were five feet ten and 125 pounds when you got married, and now you're five feet ten and 200 pounds, do you think he is not going to be pleased if you lose that weight? Sure he is. But if you tell him about your diet and then don't hit your goal, you will be letting your husband down as well as yourself. He, too, was looking forward to getting back into your size 8 pants—only in a different sense.

But that's not the worst part. The worst part is when you tell someone the secret of what you are going through and all that person does is ride you about every bite; it becomes an uphill struggle and one that is now more difficult than it would have been if you'd kept your mouth shut about the diet in the first place!

So keep your secrets to yourself and your head high. There are much better ways to torture the man in your life than to remind him of the body you once had and will probably never have again. And if you don't know what they are, write to me and I will be happy to fill you in!

## SURVIVAL HINTS

1. No one needs to know but you that you're on a diet, so keep it to yourself.
2. What's another week of torture if your diet finally works?
3. You will only wear out the rear end of your Levis if you try to shove a size 12 into a size 8.

# Dieting Deprivation

*Pamela K. Brodowsky*

**D**eprivation
**I**nsanity
**E**xcruciating
**T**orment

THAT'S WHAT *DIET* STANDS FOR!

When the word *diet* comes on the scene, the word "determination" goes out the window for me. What is the struggle here? Your mind does not tell you to consume the funnel cake at the local fair, or the Danish or other favorite pastry at the local bakery. Your mind says to your body, "You can't have that," and your body replies with a "Who the hell do you think you are, telling me what to do?" Can you really stay away from the things you really desire? Yes. Can you spell *deprivation*?

Have you ever checked to see whether someone is watching before you sneak a bite of something that looks really tasty? Do you get up for late-night snacks when everyone else is sleeping? Do you hide candy bars in your desk? Are you a closet eater?

Your mind says, "You shouldn't," but your body says, "Mind your own damn business!" Can you really make sense of these actions? *Insanity!*

How often do you torture yourself with "if onlys"? If only I were skinny. If only I could just stick to this diet. If only I could just fit back into those jeans, then I would be happy. This kind of negative self-talk is *excruciating!*

Do you buy foods for the family that you are not allowed to eat on your current diet? At the supermarket, do you purposely stop in the aisles that you know contain your "can't haves"? Do you stand and gawk in front of the bakery window? *Torment!*

All good that comes in this world comes with a price. Diets are no different. Most of the things in life we want are a gain; we want more cars, houses, money—all these things we add to our lives. Diets, on the other hand, come from something we want to lose. Fat! But we put the fat into our bodies, therefore we must take it out.

Depriving yourself constantly only hurts your chance of dieting success. Driving yourself insane with "can haves" and "can't haves" will lead only to failure. Making your life or the lives of others around you excruciating will make things more difficult for you. And tormenting yourself about what you could not accomplish is only the icing on the cake that you can't have. So be careful and treat yourself once in a while, but only in moderation.

## SURVIVAL HINTS

1. Don't deprive yourself of everything you love to eat all the time; otherwise you might end up bingeing on those very foods and treats.
2. It's only food, so don't obsess about it. Think about all the other great things in life besides eating!

# The War Within

*P. Kristen Morath*

I'M ON A DIET. I have finally come to the conclusion that I had to declare war on my own body. For years I suffered the effects as my weight went up and down: clothes that no longer fit because they were either too small or too big. There was no happy medium for me. I used to be a medium now that I think of it; however, for the last five years I haven't touched anything out of the large department. In fact, I think I might have been heading even deeper into the fat zone. I was large, larger than I had ever been in my life.

"It's *war*," I yelled to my reflection in the mirror. "You have had it. Just look at yourself. You are disgusting." And what was I going to do about it? "That's it for you, you fat-consuming blivit. I will meet you on the front lines."

That day, I emptied the refrigerator and then went on to empty every cabinet in the house. I was foodless by the end of the day, not to mention damned hungry. That evening, I made a trip to the health food store; three hundred dollars later, I refilled my cabinets and fridge with food, but only the kind that wouldn't make me fat. In fact, it was food that I was never going to eat. Food I didn't even like, and some I had never even heard of.

What the hell was I doing? I would never make it this way. My alter ego said, "Oh, yes you will." But my growling belly said, "Go get some real food." I wasn't ready to wave the white flag, but I knew I had to do something to preserve my piece of mind, save my sanity, and stick to some sort of diet that would work for me.

So rather than deprive myself of everything I wanted, I made a list of the foods I loved best. And for every three days in which I ate healthy food, I rewarded myself with a snack of food from my favorites list, but only in the portion size that could fill the palm of my hand.

Three weeks of living this way knocked twelve pounds off me. "The war is over," I declared. However, the fight had just begun.

## SURVIVAL HINTS

1. It could take many adjustments before you discover the right diet for you. But you have to start somewhere, and some kind of attempt is better than none at all.

2. Don't give in—stick to your plans and lose that fat, even if you have to keep readjusting your methods until you find out what works best for you.

# Resources

Here are some of the best sites we found for dieting information and support. There's plenty out there, so take a look around for the ones that best suit your needs.

http://www.nlm.nih.gov/medlineplus/weightlossanddieting.html

www.freedieting.com

www.weightlossforgood.co.uk

www.dietbites.com

www.weight-loss-i.com

http://www.consumer.gov/weightloss/

www.ediets.com

www.caloriescount.com

www.fitday.com

www.thedietchannel.com

http://my.webmd.com/medical_information/
condition_centers/weight_control/default.htm

http://www.thecolumn.org/

www.dietsurf.com

www.americanheart.com

www.fatlosstips.com

www.dietwatch.com

www.nutritiondata.com

www.bestofweightloss.com

www.weightwatchers.com

http://www.diet-blog.com/

http://chetday.com/dietmenu.html

# Acknowledgments

The authors would like to acknowledge the staff at Da Capo Press and to thank all the contributors to this volume for making this the best book possible. Special thanks must go to Ed Fitzgerald, Joyce Romano, and Arline Simpson, who each wrote great and funny stories for more than one volume of our Staying Sane series.